Rapid Response Situations

Rapid Response Situations

Management in Adult and Geriatric Hospitalist Medicine

GULNARA DAVUD ALIYEVA, MD, MPH

Attending Hospitalist Physician
St. Elizabeth Hospital
Appleton, WI,
United States

ELSEVIER

Elsevier
1600 John F. Kennedy Blvd.
Ste 1800
Philadelphia, PA 19103-2899

Rapid Response Situations, FIRST EDITION   ISBN: 978-0-323-83375-2
Copyright © 2022 by Elsevier, Inc. All rights reserved.

Notice

Library of Congress Control Number : 2021937495

Publisher: Dolores Meloni
Senior Content Strategist: Charlotta Kryhl
Senior Editorial Project Manager: Barbara Makinster
Production Project Manager: Poulouse Joseph
Cover Designer: Mark Rogers

Printed in India

Last digit is the print number: 9 8 7 6 5 4 3

Working together
to grow libraries in
developing countries

www.elsevier.com • www.bookaid.org

To all my patients, my father Davud, my mother Latifa, my father in law Robert, my mother in law Karen and my husband Erik.

CONTENTS

Introduction   xi

1   Cardiac Emergencies   1
Syncope   1
Acute Decompensated Heart Failure   3
Acute Coronary Syndrome   6
Cardiogenic Shock   8
Atrial Fibrillation With Rapid Ventricular Response   10
Hypertensive Emergency With Encephalopathy   13
Hypertensive Emergency With Hemorrhagic Stroke   15
Hypertensive Emergency With Acute Aortic Dissection   17
Acute Pericarditis   19
Acute Cardiac Tamponade   21

2   Respiratory Emergencies   23
Acute Asthma Exacerbation/Status Asthmaticus   23
Chronic Obstructive Pulmonary Disease (COPD) Exacerbation   26
Aspiration Pneumonitis   29
Life-Threatening Hemoptysis   31
ARDS (Acute Respiratory Distress Syndrome)   34
Massive Pulmonary Embolism   36
Severe Acute Atelectasis   39
Spontaneous Pneumothorax   41
Tension Pneumothorax   43
Acute Hypercapnic Respiratory Failure Due to Oversedation   45
Acute Partial Upper Airway Obstruction   47
Acute Complete Upper Airway Obstruction   49
Idiopathic Pulmonary Fibrosis Exacerbation   51
Acute Pulmonary Arterial Hypertension   53
Anaphylaxis   56
Acute Nonhistaminergic Angioedema   58

3   Neurological Emergencies   61
Seizure/Status Epilepticus   61
Acute Ischemic Stroke   63

Acute Hemorrhagic Stroke   66

Acute Intracranial Hypertension   69

Delirium/Agitation in Intensive Care Unit/Hospital Wards   71

Myasthenic Crisis   74

Guillain-Barre Syndrome   76

Serotonin Syndrome   79

Neuroleptic Malignant Syndrome   81

4   Gastrointestinal Emergencies   83

Upper Gastrointestinal Bleeding   83

Lower Gastrointestinal Bleeding   85

Acute Liver Failure   88

Severe Acute Pancreatitis   92

Acute Ischemic Colitis   95

Acute Mesenteric Ischemia   97

5   Endocrine Emergencies   99

Severe Diabetic Ketoacidosis   99

Hyperosmolar Hyperglycemic State   101

Hyperthyroidism/Thyroid Storm   103

Hypothryroidism/Myxedema Coma   105

Acute Adrenal (Addisonian) Crisis   107

Hypercalcemic Crisis   109

Hypocalcemic Crisis   111

Acute Severe Hypernatremia   113

Acute Severe Hyponatremia   115

Acute Severe Hyperkalemia   117

Acute Severe Hypokalemia   119

6   Hematologic Emergencies   121

Acute Blood Transfusion Reaction—Febrile Nonhemolytic
Reaction   121

Urticarial Allergic Reaction   123

Acute Blood Transfusion Reaction—Transfusion Associated Circulatory
Overload (TACO)   125

Acute Blood Transfusion Reaction—Transfusion-Related Acute Lung Injury
(TRALI)   127

Acute Blood Transfusion Reaction—Anaphylactic Reaction   129

Acute Blood Transfusion Reaction—Acute Hemolytic Reaction   131

Acute Heparin-Induced Thrombocytopenia (HIT)   133

Disseminated Intravascular Coagulation (DIC)   136

Acute Chest Syndrome in Sickle Cell Disease   138

Acute Immune Thrombocytopenia (ITP)   140

Thrombotic Thrombocytopenic Purpura (TTP)   142

Atypical Hemolytic Uremic Syndrome (HUS)   144

7   Oncologic Emergencies   147

Tumor Lysis Syndrome   147

Severe Hypercalcemia of Malignancy   149

Syndrome of Inappropriate Antidiuretic Hormone (SIADH)   151

Febrile Neutropenia   153

Acute Hyperviscosity Syndrome   155

Superior Vena Cava Syndrome   157

Malignant Epidural Spinal Cord Compression   159

Rapidly Accumulating Malignant Pericardial Effusion   161

8   Infectious Disease Emergencies   163

Sepsis and Septic Shock   163

Acute Hypoxemic Respiratory Failure Due to Severe Pneumonia   166

Hypovolemic Shock Due to Acute Infectious Diarrheal Illness   169

Acute Respiratory Failure Due to Influenza Virus Infection   172

Acute Respiratory Failure Due to COVID-19 (Coronavirus Disease of 2019) Pneumonia   175

9   Management of Postprocedural Complications in Hospitalized Patients   179

Tracheostomy Basics   179

Short-Term Tracheostomy Complication (<7 Days): Accidental Decannulation (Removal) of the Tracheostomy Tube   181

Short-Term Tracheostomy Complication (<7 Days): Tracheostomy Site Hemorrhage   182

Long-Term Tracheostomy Complication (>7 Days): Blockage of the Tracheostomy Tube   184

Long-Term Tracheostomy Complication (>7 Days): Accidental Decanulation (Removal) of the Tracheostomy Tube   186

Long-Term Tracheostomy Complication (>7 Days): Tracheo-Esophageal Fistula   188

Long-Term Tracheostomy Complication (>7 Days): Tracheo-Innominate Fistula   190

Cardiac Catheterization Complication: Hematoma at the Access Site at Common Femoral Artery   192

Cardiac Catheterization Complications: Retroperitoneal Hematoma   193

Cardiac Catheterization Complications: Contrast-Induced Nephropathy   194

Cardiac Catheterization Complications: Pseudoaneurysm, Arteriovenous Fistula, or Femoral Artery Occlusion   196

Cardiac Catheterization Complications: Anaphylactoid Reactions   198

Paracentesis Complications: Paracentesis-Induced Circulatory Dysfunction   200

Paracentesis Complications: Persistent Leakage of Ascitic Fluid From Puncture Site   201

Paracentesis Complications: Hemorrhage   202

Paracentesis Complications: Visceral Perforation (Bladder, Stomach, Bowel)   204

Complications of Thoracentesis: Pneumothorax   206

Complications of Thoracentesis: Hemothorax   208

Complications of Thoracentesis: Infection/Empyema   210

Complications of Thoracentesis: Liver/Spleen Injury   212

Complications of Lumbar Puncture: Post-LP Headache   213

Complications of Lumbar Puncture: Spinal Hematoma   214

Complications of Lumbar Puncture: Cerebral Herniation   216

10   Rapid Response Cases   219

Case I   219

Case II   221

Case III   222

Case IV   223

Case V   224

Index   225

Development of rapid response teams (RRTs) is one of the quality improvement strategies of the Institute for Healthcare Improvement, an organization founded in 1991 to increase patient safety and reduce preventable harm, errors, and delays in healthcare systems.[1] Research has shown that patients develop symptoms and signs of clinical deterioration within 6–8 h prior to a code event.[2,3] These changes may include alterations in mental status, dizziness, chest pain, and changes in vital signs. An RRT's main goal is to intervene early and prevent a patient from deteriorating to the point when code activation is necessary. Although metaanalyses of studies assessing RRTs have not consistently demonstrated that they reduce in-hospital morbidity or mortality, many healthcare systems in developed countries have implemented RRTs as a standard of care. The 2008 Joint Commission on Accreditation of Healthcare Organizations (JCAHO) requires the implementation of RRTs.

The most common criteria for rapid response team activation are:

- threatened airway
- acute change in RR < 8 or > 28 per min
- acute change in oxygen saturation < 90% despite oxygen supplementation
- acute change in heart rate < 40 or > 140 bpm
- acute change in systolic BP < 90 mmHg
- acute change in consciousness
- urine output less than 50 cc over 4 h
- chest pain unrelieved by nitroglycerin
- seizure
- staff member has significant concern about the patient's condition

The typical rapid response team usually includes:

- hospitalist or intensivist (to evaluate the patient, order laboratory tests and medications, coordinate team efforts, make patient triage decisions)
- ICU RN (to assess IV access, manage crash cart, administer medications)
- respiratory therapist (to manage airway, such as administer oxygen, set up suction, ventilate the patient with a bag-valve mask, initiate BiPAP)
- pharmacist (to prepare medications)
- phlebotomist (to draw blood for laboratory tests)

This pocket book is intended for hospitalists who are increasingly assuming RRT duties and for all members of rapid response teams; its purpose is to enable quick assessments and stabilization of acutely ill patients. In a step-by-step fashion, this pocket book addresses most common rapid response situations and provides guidance on how to effectively manage critically ill patients. The concise format of the text provides quick access to the information most needed at the time of an emergency, including which stabilization measures to implement, which tests to order, which specialists to consult, and the dosage of medications.

References

1. *5 Million Lives Campaign. Getting Started Kit: Rapid Response Teams.* Cambridge, MA: Institute for Healthcare Improvement; 2008.
2. Schein RM, Hazday N, Pena M, et al. Clinical antecedents to in-hospital cardiopulmonary arrest. *Chest.* 1990;98:1388–1392.
3. Franklin C, Mathew J. Developing strategies to prevent in hospital cardiac arrest: analyzing responses of physicians and nurses in the hours before the event. *Crit Care Med.* 1994;22(2):244–247.

CHAPTER 1

Cardiac Emergencies

Syncope

Presentation

Transient self-limited loss of consciousness and inability to maintain postural tone, excluding seizure, shock, or coma.[1] Causes of syncope can range from benign to life-threatening.

Types of syncope:

Vasovagal (neurocardiogenic) syncope, the most common and the most benign type of syncope	*Cardiac syncope*	*Neurologic syncope*
Postural (orthostatic) hypotension	Arrhythmia (tachy-and brady-arrhythmias)	Seizure
Dehydration	Myocardial infarction	Stroke
Postprandial	Valvular heart disease	TIA (transient ischemic attack)
Blood draw	(for example, aortic valve stenosis)	Vertebrobasilar insufficiency
Intense emotional stress	Congestive heart failure	
Pain	HOCM (hypertrophic obstructive cardiomyopathy)	
Forceful cough	Pulmonary embolism	
Carotid sinus hypersensitivity (turning the neck, tight collar, shaving the neck area)		
Urinating (micturition)		
Defecation		
Hyperventilation		
Alcohol/drugs		

Many patients may have premonitory symptoms such as dizziness, lightheadedness, blacking out, feeling unsteady and weak, and vision changes such as seeing stars and spots, tunnel vision, or nausea.

Causes for Rapid Response Activation

Syncope, hypotension, tachycardia.

Actions

INITIAL MEASURES

1. Continuous pulse oximetry
2. Supplemental oxygen to maintain $SpO_2 > 92\%$
3. Continuous cardiac monitoring/blood pressure measurements

DIAGNOSTIC WORK-UP

1. History and physical exam are the most sensitive and specific ways to evaluate syncope and its precipitating factors.
2. 12-Lead EKG may show acute MI, cardiac ischemia, arrhythmia, bradycardia, tachycardia, atrioventricular blocks, and pauses; compare to prior EKGs.
3. Rapid fingerstick to check blood glucose level.
4. Labs: CBC (acute blood loss anemia), BMP (electrolyte abnormalities, e.g., hyponatremia due to diuretic use), troponin (especially if patient has exertional syncope, chest pain, or dyspnea), CK (elevated after seizure), BNP, TSH, UA (UTI, especially in elderly patients), and stool guaiac (if patient is anemic).
5. Orthostatic vital signs after the patient is stabilized.
6. If patient has a pacemaker, it will have to be interrogated by a manufacturer.
7. Chest X-ray (pneumonia, pulmonary edema, pleural effusions, widened mediastinum).
8. Noncontrast CT scan of head (in patients with new neurological deficits, trauma due to syncope, hydrocephalus).
9. Echocardiogram (test of choice for evaluation of cardiac syncope; can identify if patient has aortic stenosis).
10. CTA of chest and abdomen, if you suspect pulmonary embolism, aortic dissection, or ruptured aortic aneurysm.
11. MRI/MRA of brain/neck in select patients.
12. EEG (electroencephalography) in select patients.
13. Stress test for patients with cardiac syncope.
14. Head-up tilt-table test to confirm autonomic dysfunction.

Treatment

1. Treat dehydration with intravenous fluids.
2. Reduce antihypertensive medications and diuretics doses.
3. Postural hypotension is treated with support garments/compression stockings, calf exercises, and drinking Gatorade; if these measures do not help, consider the following options:
   - Midodrine 2.5–10 mg PO q 8h[2]
   - Fludrocortisone (Florinef) 0.1 mg PO daily[3]
4. Treat arrhythmias with antiarrhythmic medications.
5. Consult electrophysiologist for consideration of pacemaker placement, if indicated.
6. Consult interventional cardiologist and cardiothoracic surgeon for consideration of corrective intervention for valvular disease.

References

1. Walsh K, Hoffmayer K, Hamdan MH. Syncope: diagnosis and management. *Curr Probl Cardiol.* 2015;40(2):51–86.
2. *Midodrine.* Reference.medscape.com.
3. *Fludrocortisone.* Reference.medscape.com.

Acute Decompensated Heart Failure

Presentation

Acute decompensated heart failure (ADHF) refers to rapid onset of fluid volume overload. The most common causes are medication and dietary noncompliance; however, acute coronary syndrome, arrhythmias, uncontrolled hypertension, and infections such as endocarditis may also cause acute decompensated heart failure.

Symptoms of acute decompensated heart failure include fatigue, cough, dyspnea, orthopnea, paroxysmal nocturnal dyspnea, weight gain, and increased abdominal girth. On physical examination, patients may have elevated jugular venous pressure, hepatojugular reflex, third heart sound, pulmonary crackles, peripheral edema, ascites, hepatomegaly, and splenomegaly.

Causes for Rapid Response Activation

Persistently worsening dyspnea, hypoxia, arrhythmias, hemodynamic instability.

Actions

INITIAL MEASURES

1. Continuous pulse oximetry
2. Supplemental oxygen to maintain $SpO_2 > 92\%$
3. Continuous cardiac monitoring

DIAGNOSTIC WORK-UP

1. Labs: CBC, BNP (> 500 in cardiogenic pulmonary edema, both diagnostic and prognostic test), troponin, BMP (to assess renal function and electrolyte abnormalities), liver function tests (will be elevated due to decreased cardiac output and increased venous congestion), and TSH.
2. EKG (may identify potential triggers for ADHF such as atrial flutter/fibrillation with rapid ventricular response or ischemia).
3. Chest X-ray (will demonstrate pulmonary vascular congestion, interstitial/alveolar edema, pleural effusion).
4. Bedside (point-of-care) ultrasound, if available (will demonstrate 3–6 bilateral "B-lines" or "comet tails").
5. STAT echocardiography in patients with hemodynamic instability/cardiogenic shock (may identify free myocardial wall rupture, ventricular septal defect, acute mitral valve regurgitation, thrombosis, pericardial tamponade, etc.).

TREATMENT

1. Bolus doses of IV furosemide 1–2.5 times the home oral dose (significant reduction in left and right ventricular filling pressures 15 min after the dose and peak effect at 1–2 h); if patient is not on a home diuretic (diuretic-naïve patient), initial dose of furosemide is 20–40 mg IV.[1]

2. Bumetanide and torsemide are equally potent alternatives to furosemide:
   - Bumetanide 1 mg IV (initial dose)
   - Torsemide 10–20 mg IV (initial dose)[1]

3. Continuous infusion of furosemide starting at 5 mg/h; titrate to 20 mg/h, if patient has inadequate response to maximum bolus dose of furosemide.[1]

4. In patients with significant fluid overload/anasarca and inability to achieve sufficient diuresis without unacceptable degree of azotemia, consult nephrologist for hemodialysis[2]; other indications for hemodialysis include oliguria, severe hyperkalemia ($K > 6.5$), and severe acidemia (pH < 7.2).

5. In patients with absence of hypotension, presence of ischemia (chest pain), presence of hypertension, or who are unresponsive to initial diuretics, administer:
   - Nitroglycerin 0.4 mg sublingually, followed by
   - Nitroglycerin drip starting at 10–20 µg/min, increase by 5–10 µg/min q 5–10 min, up to 60 µg/min, maximum dose 200–500 µg/min[3]

6. Noninvasive positive pressure ventilation (NIPPV) in patients with adequate airway protection, BiPAP is preferred.[4]

7. Invasive positive pressure ventilation (PPV) in patients with progressive hypoxia despite optimal use of noninvasive respiratory support or with inadequate airway protection; initial ventilator setting in patients with ADHF with reduced ejection fraction:
   - Mode of ventilation: assist control.
   - Initial FiO_2: 100%; once patient stabilizes, titrate down to maintain SpO_2 at 90%–94%.
   - PEEP: 5 cmH$_2$O.
   - Tidal volume (VT) 6–8 mL/kg of predicted (ideal) body weight:
     - Male: PBW (kg) = 50 + 2.3(height(in)-60)
     - Female: PBW (kg) = 45.5 + 2.3(height(in)-60)
   - RR: 10–12 breaths per minute; titrate to maintain normal pH of 7.35–7.45.
   - Inspiratory to expiratory ratio I/E of 1:2.
   - Maintain plateau pressure (Pplat) ≤ 30 cmH$_2$O to avoid barotrauma.
   - Monitor clinical response, Pplat, and ABGs closely.[5]

8. In patients with decreased cardiac output such as hypotension (sBP < 80) due to hypoperfusion (cool/clammy legs, obtunded, decreased urine output), elevated cardiac filling pressures (elevated JVP on exam), or worsening renal function, start one of the following options:
   - Dobutamine starting at 0.5–1 µg/kg/min; may titrate up to 2–20 µg/kg/min.
   - Milrinone starting at 0.1 µg/kg/min; titrate up to 0.2–0.3 µg/kg/min, maximum dose 0.75 µg/kg/min.

   These patients will likely need invasive hemodynamic monitoring (e.g., pulmonary artery catheter).[2]

9. Identify and treat precipitating factors (e.g., atrial fibrillation, myocardial ischemia, thyroid disorder, etc.).

References

1. Felker GM. Diuretic strategies in patients with acute decompensated heart failure (DOSE study). *N Engl J Med.* 2011;364:797–805.
2. Evaluation and management of patients with acute decompensated heart failure. *J Cardiac Fail.* 2010;16(6):e134–e156.
3. Elkayam U. IV nitroglycerin in the treatment of decompensated heart failure: potential benefits and limitations. *J Cardiovasc Pharmacol Ther.* 2004;9:227–241.
4. Gray AJ. 3CPO Study Investigators. A multicenter randomized controlled trial of the use of continuous positive airway pressure and non-invasive positive pressure ventilation in the early treatment of patients presenting to the emergency department with severe acute cardiogenic pulmonary edema. *Health Technol Assess.* 2009;13:1–106.
5. Kuhn B. Management of mechanical ventilation in decompensated heart failure. *J Cardiovasc Devel Dis.* 2016;3(4):33.

Acute Coronary Syndrome

Presentation

Acute coronary syndrome is caused by a blockage of the coronary artery from cholesterol-rich plaque and thrombus. Symptoms include chest pain, tightness, fullness, pressure, or other anginal equivalents, including pain in arms, jaw, neck, back, or abdomen, shortness of breath, dizziness, nausea, indigestion, or diaphoresis.

Partially obstructive coronary occlusion without cardiac injury (normal troponin) is unstable angina (UA). Partially obstructive coronary occlusion with cardiac injury (elevated troponin > 0.08) is non-ST elevation acute coronary syndrome (NSTE-ACS). In ST elevation myocardial infarction (STEMI), atherothrombotic plaque leads to total occlusion of the coronary artery with complete cessation of blood flow.

Causes for Rapid Response Activation

Persistently worsening chest pain and other anginal equivalents.

Actions

INITIAL MEASURES

1. Continuous pulse oximetry
2. Supplemental oxygen to maintain $SpO_2 > 92\%$
3. Continuous cardiac monitoring
4. Consultation with cardiologist early in the course of illness

DIAGNOSTIC WORK-UP

1. 12-Lead EKG within 10 min of onset allows identification of STEMI: ST-segment elevation ≥ 1 mm in at least two contiguous leads.
2. Cardiac troponin is the preferred biomarker of myocardial injury; check troponin at onset (may be normal initially) and every 3–6 h after onset of symptoms.
3. Other labs: CBC, coagulations studies (INR, PT, aPTT), BMP, and magnesium.
4. Echocardiography may be useful in patients with UA/NSTE-ACS, as it may show regional wall motion abnormalities and identify involved coronary territory.

TREATMENT

1. STEMI is treated with primary percutaneous coronary intervention (PPCI); door to balloon time < 90 min.
2. If no PPCI is available at the hospital, transport the patient to a hospital with PPCI capacity if the total door to balloon time, including transport, will be less than 120 min.

3. If the total door to balloon time, including transport, will be > 120 min, treat patient with fibrinolytic therapy, such as alteplase, if there are no contraindications, within 30 min from the onset of symptoms, and then transport patient to a hospital with PPCI capacity in case fibrinolysis does not work or the patient develops recurrent infarction.

4. In patients with NSTE-ACS/UA, do early risk stratification, for example, using TIMI or GRACE risk score to identify low- and high-risk patients.

5. Low-risk patients will need serial troponins; if serial troponins are normal, the next step will be stress testing; if serial troponins are abnormal, the next step will be coronary angiography.

6. Administer nitroglycerin 0.4 mg sublingually every 5 min up to three times for patients with chest pain.

7. If chest pain persists, start nitroglycerin drip at 5–10 µg/min; titrate up by 10 µg/min every 10 min, until resolution of chest pain or systolic BP < 100 mmHg (nitrates are contraindicated in patients who took phosphodiesterase III inhibitors for erectile dysfunction within 48 h or sBP < 90 mmHg).

8. Administer aspirin 162–325 mg orally (chew to enhance absorption) or rectally.

9. Additional antiplatelet options—discuss with cardiologist:
   - Clopidogrel loading dose of 300–600 mg orally once, then 75 mg daily; should be held 5 days prior to CABG.
   - Ticagrelor 180 mg orally once, then 90 mg orally twice daily; should be held 5 days prior to CABG.
   - Prasugrel 60 mg orally once, then 10 mg orally daily; patients < 60 kg or > 75 years may use 5 mg orally daily; contraindicated in patients with prior CVA, including TIA; prasugrel should be held 7 days prior to CABG.
   - Heparin IV drip.

10. Oral beta-blocker in patients without hypotension, heart block, bradycardia, or decompensated systolic dysfunction.
    - Metoprolol succinate 25–200 mg orally daily.

11. Angiotensin converting enzyme inhibitor in patients with left ventricular ejection fraction of ≤ 40%, without evidence of hypotension, shock, or bilateral renal artery stenosis.
    - Lisinopril 5–40 mg orally daily.

12. Atorvastatin 80 mg orally daily.

13. Morphine 1–4 mg IV; repeat every 2–6 h as needed for chest pain, while monitoring oxygen saturation/blood pressure.

Further Reading

1. Amsterdam EA, Wenger NK, Brindis RG, et al. AHA/ACC guideline for the management of patients with non–ST-elevation acute coronary syndromes: a report of the American College of Cardiology/American Heart Association Task Force on Practice Guidelines. *J Am Coll Cardiol.* 2014;64(24):e139–e228.

Cardiogenic Shock

Presentation

Cardiogenic shock is a low cardiac output state that leads to end-organ hypoperfusion and hypoxia associated with multiorgan failure. Morbidity and mortality associated with cardiogenic shock remain high.

The most frequent cause of cardiogenic shock is acute myocardial infarction with left ventricular dysfunction.[1] Other causes include acute decompensated heart failure, acute myocarditis, stress-induced cardiomyopathy, advanced valvular heart disease, and postcardiotomy shock in patient with recent cardiac surgery.

Clinical criteria include systolic blood pressure < 90 mmHg for ≥ 30 min, pulmonary congestion, and evidence of end-organ hypoperfusion, such as altered mental status, cold/clammy skin and extremities, sinus tachycardia, urine output < 30 mL/h, or lactate > 2 mmol/L.[2]

Causes for Rapid Response Activation

Progressively worsening hypoxia and hemodynamic instability.

Actions

INITIAL MEASURES

1. Continuous pulse oximetry
2. Supplemental oxygen to maintain SpO_2 > 92% or PaO_2 > 60 mmHg
3. Continuous cardiac monitoring
4. Consultation with cardiologist and cardiovascular surgeon early in the course of illness

DIAGNOSTIC WORK-UP

1. 12-Lead EKG within 10 min of onset of symptoms.[3]
2. Transthoracic echocardiography to identify the cause of the cardiogenic shock and to assess mechanical complications of acute coronary syndrome, such as papillary muscle rupture, ventricular septal defect, free myocardial wall rupture, or pericardial tamponade.[4]
3. Labs: serial troponins, BNP, lactic acid (elevated in tissue hypoxia and associated with higher mortality), CBC, BMP, magnesium, liver transaminases (elevated in liver hypoperfusion injury), and ABG (arterial blood gas).
4. Chest X-ray to allow assessment of cardiac size, widened mediastinum, pulmonary congestion, or pleural effusion.

TREATMENT

1. Place central line for volume resuscitation and multiple medication infusions.
2. Place arterial line for continuous blood pressure monitoring.

3. Invasive hemodynamic monitoring such as pulmonary artery catheterization to exclude other types of shock, such as hypovolemic or septic shock, and the hemodynamic measurements of cardiogenic shock: pulmonary capillary wedge pressure (PCWP) > 15 mmHg and a cardiac index (CI) < 2.2 L/min/m.[2]

4. Pulmonary artery catheterization may also be indicative of RV infarction (high right-side filling pressures in the absence of an elevated PCWP), severe mitral valve regurgitation (large V wave on the PCWP tracing), or ventricular septal rupture (step up in oxygen saturation between right atrium and right ventricle).[5]

5. If no evidence of fluid overload exists, proceed with IV fluid resuscitation with normal saline as a first-line treatment.

6. Administer vasopressors for hemodynamic support to maintain MAP of 60–65 mmHg:
   - Dopamine 5–10 μg/kg/min IV; titrate up to 20 μg/kg/min.[6]
   - If patient remains hypotensive, add norepinephrine 0.2 μg/kg/min; titrate up to 3.3 μg/kg/min.[7]

7. Inotropes to decrease afterload and increase cardiac output:
   - Dobutamine in a range of 2–20 μg/kg/min[8]
   - Milrinone in a range of 0.3–0.75 μg/kg/min[9]

8. Correct electrolyte abnormalities such as hypokalemia and hypomagnesemia.

9. Consider continuous renal replacement therapy in patients with serum creatinine ≥ 2.0 times baseline and urine output < 0.5 mL/kg/h for ≥ 12 h.[1]

10. Start intubation and mechanical ventilation for patients with worsening hypoxia or inadequate airway protection.

11. In patients with acute coronary syndrome, consult cardiologist for coronary reperfusion such as PCI/fibrinolysis; consult cardiovascular surgeon for patients who will likely require CABG.

12. Patients may need temporary mechanical circulatory support such as IABP (intra-aortic balloon pump), ECMO (extracorporeal membrane oxygenation), or peripheral/implantable VAD (ventricular assist device).

References

1. Van Diepen S, et al. Contemporary management of cardiogenic shock: a scientific statement from the American Heart Association. *Circulation.* 2017;136:e232–e268.

2. Thiele H, et al. IABP-SHOCK II trial investigator. Intraaortic balloon support for myocardial infarction with cardiogenic shock. *N Engl J Med.* 2012;367:1287–1296.

3. Amsterdam EA, Wenger NK, Brindis RG, et al. AHA/ACC guideline for the management of patients with non–ST-elevation acute coronary syndromes: a report of the American College of Cardiology/American Heart Association Task Force on Practice Guidelines. *J Am Coll Cardiol.* 2014;64(24):e139–e228.

4. Kutty RS, Jones N, Moorjani N. Mechanical complications of acute myocardial infarction. *Cardiol Clin.* 2013;31:519–531.

5. O'Gara PT, et al. 2013 ACCF/AHA guideline for the management of ST-elevation myocardial infarction. *Circulation.* 2013;127:e362–e425.

6. Dopamine. Reference.medscape.com.

7. Norepinephrine. Reference.medscape.com.

8. Dobutamine. Reference.medscape.com.

9. Milrinone. Reference.medscape.com.

Atrial Fibrillation With Rapid Ventricular Response

Presentation

Atrial fibrillation with rapid ventricular response is common among patients with critical illnesses. It is associated with increased morbidity and mortality. Diagnosis of atrial fibrillation is confirmed by a 12-lead EKG. Obesity and obstructive sleep apnea are the most important risk factors for atrial fibrillation.[1]

Patients may be asymptomatic. Common symptoms include fatigue, palpitations, angina, dyspnea, orthopnea, dizziness, or syncope. On physical examination, patient will be tachycardic with irregularly irregular pulse and may have rales on pulmonary auscultation. Atrial fibrillation with rapid ventricular response may be associated with tachycardia-induced cardiomyopathy or systemic thromboembolism.

Causes for Rapid Response Activation

Moderate to severe symptoms of atrial fibrillations, such as palpitations, dyspnea, dizziness, angina.

Actions

INITIAL MEASURES

1. Continuous pulse oximetry
2. Supplemental oxygen to maintain $SpO_2 > 92\%$
3. Continuous cardiac monitoring

DIAGNOSTIC WORK-UP

1. 12-Lead EKG: replacement of P waves with fibrillatory waves with irregular narrow QRS with rapid ventricular heart rate 110–170 bpm.
2. Labs: CBC, BMP, magnesium, TSH, troponin, BNP, and D-dimer.
3. Echocardiogram to allow evaluation of valvular disease, atrial and ventricular chamber size, left ventricular function, left ventricular hypertrophy, pulmonary hypertension, and pericardial disease.

TREATMENT

1. Lenient rate control with heart rate < 110 bpm on ECG is sufficient to improve atrial fibrillation–related symptoms.[1]
2. Use first-line agents for rate control to achieve target heart rate < 110 bpm:
   - Metoprolol as IV boluses 2.5–5.0 mg over 2 min; repeat at 5-min intervals with close monitoring of blood pressure until target heart rate is achieved.[2]

- Esmolol; start with bolus 500 µg/kg over 1 min, followed by 50 µg/kg/min; increase by 50 µg/kg/min every 5–30 min to a maximum dose of 200 µg/kg/min; acts rapidly, with a short half-life; useful in patients with marginal hemodynamic stability.[2]
- Diltiazem IV bolus of 0.25 mg/kg (average 20 mg) over 2 min; if the first bolus is tolerated but does not achieve target heart rate, a second bolus of 0.35 mg/kg (average 25 mg) can be given 10–15 min after the first bolus, followed by an infusion at a rate of 5–15 mg/h.[2]
- Verapamil 5–10 mg IV over 2 min, followed by a maintenance infusion rate of approximately 0.125 mg/min; bolus dose can be repeated every 15–30 min as needed.[2]

3. Digoxin may be added as a second agent in patients with heart failure with reduced left ventricular ejection fraction; use with caution in elderly patients and patients with renal failure:
   - Slow oral digitalization: 0.125–0.25 mg orally daily; in patients with moderate to severe renal failure: 0.0625 mg daily or 0.125 mg every other day, to avoid digoxin toxicity.[2]
   - Rapid IV digitalization: 0.25–0.5 mg IV over several min, followed by 0.25 mg every 4–6 h until a total of 0.75–1.5 mg has been given.[2]
   - Rapid oral digitalization: 0.5 mg orally, followed by 0.25–0.5 mg every 6 h until a total of 0.75–1.5 mg has been given.[2]

4. Amiodarone can be used in patients with no accessory pathway when other measures are unsuccessful or contraindicated, with dosage of 150 mg IV over 10 min, followed by a maintenance dose of 0.5–1 mg/min IV.[2]

5. Administer magnesium 2.5 g over 20 min, followed by 2.5 g over 2 h.[2]

6. Assess stroke risk with CHA_2DS_2-VASc score (CHF, HTN, age ≥ 75, diabetes, stroke/TIA/thromboembolism, vascular disease such as MI, PAD, or aortic plaque, age 65–74, sex category: female).[3]

7. Assess hemorrhage risk with HAS-BLED score (hypertension, abnormal renal function and liver function, stroke, prior major bleeding, labile INR, elderly > 65 years, drugs predisposing to bleeding and alcohol); if HAS-BLED score is ≥ 3, patient has a high risk for hemorrhage.[1]

8. Antiplatelets (e.g., aspirin) alone are no longer recommended for patients with low CHA_2DS_2-VASc scores.[1,3]

9. If CHA_2DS_2-VASc score is 1 in men or 2 in women, NOACs can be *considered*.[1,3]

10. If CHA_2DS_2-VASc score is ≥ 2 in men or ≥ 3 in women, NOACs are *recommended* over warfarin except in patients with moderate-to-severe mitral stenosis or a mechanical heart valve, for whom warfarin is recommended[1,3]:
    - Apixaban 5 mg orally twice daily; 2.5 mg orally twice daily for patients with ≥ 2 of the following: creatinine > 1.5 mg/dL, age > 80, weight < 132 lb (60 kg).
    - Rivaroxaban 20 mg orally daily; 15 mg daily for CrCl 15–50 mL/min/1.73 m²; not recommended if CrCl < 15 mL/min/1.73 m².
    - Dabigatran 150 mg orally twice daily; 75 mg orally twice daily for CrCl 15–30 mL/min/1.73 m²; not recommended if CrCl < 15 mL/min/1.73 m².
    - Edoxaban 60 mg orally daily; 30 mg daily if CrCl 15–50 mL/min/1.73 m²; avoid use if CrCl > 95 mL/min/1.73 m² due to increased clearance; not recommended if CrCl < 15 mL/min/1.73 m²; avoid in Child-Pugh Class B or C liver disease.[4]

11. Request a cardiology consultation regarding rhythm control, such as nonemergent cardioversion, for patients with poorly tolerated atrial fibrillation that is refractory to drug therapy to improve symptoms and quality of life.

12. Nonemergent cardioversion may be considered if duration of atrial fibrillation is < 48 h.

13. If duration of atrial fibrillation is unknown, one of the following options may be considered:
    ■ Anticoagulate for 3 weeks before and 4 weeks after cardioversion
    ■ Transesophageal (TEE)-guided cardioversion; that is, start NOAC ≥ 4h before cardioversion, cardiovert if TEE shows no evidence of thrombus in cardiac chambers, especially in left atrial appendage[5]
14. Consider catheter ablation in patients with symptomatic atrial fibrillation and heart failure with reduced left ventricular ejection fraction (HFrEF) to reduce mortality rate and rate of hospitalization for heart failure.[3]
15. Percutaneous left atrial appendage (LAA) occlusion (Watchman device) may be considered for patients with atrial fibrillation and increased risk for stroke and who have contraindications to long-term anticoagulation.[3]
16. For management of atrial fibrillation in hemodynamically unstable patients, please follow Advanced Cardiac Life Support (ACLS) protocol.

References

1. Crawford TC. *ESC Guidelines for Atrial Fibrillation: Key Points*; 2020. Acc.org.
2. Stambler B, Zavaneh M. *Atrial Fibrillation: Rate Control: Options, Advantages, Disadvantages*; 2013. Thecardiologyadvisor.com.
3. January CT, Wann LS, Calkins H, et al. 2019 AHA/ACC/HRS focused update of the 2014 AHA/ACC/HRS guideline for the management of patients with atrial fibrillation: a report of the American College of Cardiology/American Heart Association Task Force on Clinical Practice. Guidelines and the Heart Rhythm Society in Collaboration With the Society of Thoracic Surgeons. *Circulation*. 2019;140:e125–e151.
4. Gutierrez C, Blanchard DC. Diagnosis and treatment of atrial fibrillation. *Am Fam Physician*. 2016;94(6):442–452.
5. Goette A, Heidbuchel H. Practical implementation of anticoagulation strategy for patients undergoing cardioversion of atrial fibrillation. *Arrhythm Electrophysiol Rev*. 2017;6(2):50–54.

Hypertensive Emergency With Encephalopathy

Presentation

Hypertensive emergency is defined as systolic blood pressure ≥ 180 mmHg or diastolic blood pressure ≥ 120 mmHg plus acute target organ damage, such as cerebral edema.[1] The most common cause is poorly controlled primary hypertension.

Hypertensive encephalopathy is manifested by headache, nausea, vomiting, lethargy, confusion, blurred vision and ultimately seizures and coma, if untreated. MRI of the head would demonstrate reversible white matter changes referred to as posterior reversible encephalopathy syndrome (PRES).

Patients with hypertensive encephalopathy may also have symptoms related to other organ damage, such as kidney damage (acute kidney injury, hematuria, proteinuria), cardiac damage (congestive heart failure) or retinal damage (papilledema, retinal hemorrhage).

Causes for Rapid Response Activation

Progressively worsening altered mental status and seizures.

Actions

INITIAL MEASURES

1. Continuous pulse oximetry
2. Supplemental oxygen to maintain $SpO_2 > 92\%$
3. Continuous cardiac monitoring
4. Continuous blood pressure monitoring

DIAGNOSTIC WORK-UP

1. Labs: CBC, peripheral blood smear, BMP, magnesium, UA (hematuria, proteinuria, casts), urine pregnancy test, and urine toxicologic screen.
2. Order noncontrast head CT scan to rule out hemorrhagic stroke or cerebral edema.
3. Renal ultrasound or echocardiography may be useful for evaluation of other organ complications.
4. Consider head MRI when patient is stable to further assess PRES or other complications.
5. Rule out causes for possible secondary hypertension when patient is stable.

TREATMENT

1. Initial goal blood pressure reduction is 10% within first hour, then, if the patient is clinically stable, by 15% more over the following 7 h, and then cautiously to normal over the following 24–48 h, to avoid ischemic stroke.[2]

2. Start a titratable agent such as:
   - Nicardipine 5 mg/h; increase by 2.5 mg/h every 15 min to maximum of 15 mg/h.
   - Clevidipine 1–2 mg/h; titrate every 90 s by doubling the dose; as the BP approaches its goal, increase the dose by less than doubling every 5–10 min, maximum dose 21 mg/h.
   - Labetalol 10–20 mg IV bolus, followed by 1–2 mg/min, maximum dose 300 mg over 24 h.
   - Esmolol, loading dose of 500 μg/kg over 1 min, followed by 25 μg/kg/min; titrate to maximum of 200 μg/kg/min.
   - Fenoldopam 0.1–0.3 μg/kg/min; titrate by 0.1 μg/kg/min every 15 min to maximum of 1.6 μg/kg/min.[3]

References

1. Arbe G, Pastor I, Franco J. Diagnostic and therapeutic approach to the hypertensive crisis. *Med Clin (Barc)*. 2018;150(8):317–322.
2. Anderson CS, et al. Intensive blood pressure reduction in acute cerebral hemorrhage trial (INTERACT): a randomized pilot trial. *Lancet Neurol*. 2008;7(5):391–399.
3. Aronow WS. Treatment of hypertensive emergencies. *Ann Transl Med*. 2017;5(1):S5.

Hypertensive Emergency With Hemorrhagic Stroke

Presentation

Hypertensive emergency is defined as systolic blood pressure ≥ 180 mmHg or diastolic blood pressure ≥ 120 mmHg plus acute target organ damage, such as hemorrhagic stroke. Hemorrhage growth is associated with increased mortality and morbidity. Patient will present with headache, nausea, vomiting, and confusion. Physical examination may show focal neurological signs such as hemiparesis, hemisensory loss, gaze preference, nystagmus, visual field cut, aphasia, or neglect.[1]

Causes for Rapid Response Activation

Progressively worsening altered mental state, stroke symptoms, or seizures.

Actions

INITIAL MEASURES

1. Continuous pulse oximetry
2. Supplemental oxygen to maintain $SpO_2 > 92\%$
3. Continuous cardiac monitoring
4. Continuous blood pressure monitoring
5. Elevation of the head of the bed to 30 degrees to improve jugular venous outflow and decrease intracranial pressure
6. Completion of a structured examination, such as the National Institute of Health (NIH) stroke scale
7. Transfer of patient to ICU or stroke unit
8. Consultation with neurosurgeon early in the course of rapid response

DIAGNOSTIC WORK-UP

1. Labs: CBC, BMP, magnesium, coagulation studies (INR, PT, aPTT) especially in patients taking anticoagulants, troponin; urine toxicology screen (cocaine); urinalysis; urine pregnancy test in women of childbearing age.
2. EKG (arrhythmias, concomitant myocardial ischemia/infarct).
3. Noncontrast CT scan of head or MRI.

TREATMENT

1. Acute BP reduction to target systolic BP of 140 mmHg early in the treatment of patients with intracerebral hemorrhage lessens the absolute growth of hematomas, particularly in patients who have received previous antithrombotic therapy, and is associated with better functional recovery.[2]

2. Start a titratable agent such as:
   - Nicardipine 5 mg/h; increase by 2.5 mg/h every 15 min to maximum of 15 mg/h.
   - Labetalol 10–20 mg IV bolus, followed by 1–2 mg/min to maximum of 300 mg over 24 h.
   - Esmolol, with loading dose of 500 µg/kg over 1 min, followed by 25 µg/kg/min; titrate to maximum of 200 µg/kg/min.[3]

3. Stop/reverse all anticoagulation[2]:
   - If patient is on warfarin, administer:
     - Vitamin K 5–10 mg IV (requires 6 h to normalize INR)
     - FFP (fresh frozen plasma) 15–20 mL/kg or PCC (prothrombin complex concentrate)

4. Transfuse platelets[2] if platelet count $< 50 \times 10^9$/L.

5. Closely monitor glucose; avoid hypoglycemia/hyperglycemia.[2]

6. If patient has seizure:
   - Check fingerstick glucose.
   - Administer lorazepam 2–4 mg IV over 2 min (if no IV access is available, midazolam 10 mg IM or diazepam 20 mg PR); may repeat lorazepam 2–4 mg IV in 5 min if necessary.
   - Follow with phenytoin 20 mg/kg IV or fosphenytoin 15–20 mg PE/kg administered at 100–150 mg PE/min or levetiracetam 500 mg IV q 12 h for longer-term control if available.
   - If seizure is not terminated within 20–25 min, administer propofol 1–2 mg/kg IV bolus, followed by 50–75 µg/kg/min and intubate.
   - Order EEG monitoring.[2]

7. Use antacids to prevent gastric ulcers associated with intracerebral hemorrhage.

8. Monitor and treat intracranial pressure (ICP) in the following situations:
   - Glasgow Coma Score (GCS) ≤ 8
   - Transtentorial herniation
   - Significant intraventricular hemorrhage or hydrocephalus[2]

9. Evacuation of hematoma is recommended in the following situations:
   - Hematoma > 3 cm in diameter
   - Cerebellar hemorrhage and neurological deterioration
   - Brainstem compression from ventricular obstruction
   - Hydrocephalus from ventricular obstruction[2]
     Evacuation can be done via open craniotomy; endovascular therapy using coil embolization can be considered.

References

1. Wajngarten M, Silva GS. Hypertension and stroke: update on treatment. *Eur Cardiol.* 2019;14(2):11–115.
2. Hemphill 3rd JC, et al. Guidelines for the management of spontaneous intracerebral hemorrhage: a guideline for healthcare professionals from the American Heart Association/American Stroke Association. *Stroke.* 2015;46(7):2032–2060.
3. Aronow WS. Treatment of hypertensive emergencies. *Ann Transl Med.* 2017;5(1):S5.

Hypertensive Emergency With Acute Aortic Dissection

Presentation

Acute aortic dissection is defined as a separation within the layers of the aortic wall that occurs within < 2 weeks from the onset of the tear.[1] This condition can be rapidly fatal in the majority of patients. Conditions that can increase aortic wall stress include uncontrolled hypertension, pheochromocytoma, coarctation of aorta, and stimulants, such as cocaine.[2] Patients with family history of aortic dissection, thoracic aortic aneurysm, personal history of aortic valve disease, recent aortic interventions, Marfan syndrome, Turner syndrome, or Ehlers-Danlos syndrome are at higher risk for aortic dissection.[2]

Symptoms of aortic dissection may include sudden onset of severe chest pain with a tearing, ripping, or stabbing quality with maximal severity at the onset of the pain; and upper back pain, syncope, dyspnea, symptoms of stroke such as hemiplegia or hemiparesis, altered mental status, Horner syndrome (ptosis, myosis, and anhidrosis), hemoptysis, anxiety, and premonition of death. On physical exam patients may have interarm blood pressure difference > 20 mmHg, bounding pulses, wide pulse pressure, diastolic murmurs, such as new aortic regurgitation murmur and focal neurological deficits.[3]

Causes for Rapid Response Activation

Progressively worsening symptoms of chest pain, stroke-like symptoms, dyspnea, altered mental state, or syncope.

Actions

INITIAL MEASURES

1. Continuous pulse oximetry
2. Supplemental oxygen to maintain SpO_2 > 92% or PaO_2 > 60 mmHg
3. Continuous cardiac monitoring
4. Continuous blood pressure monitoring
5. Two large-bore IV lines
6. Transfer of patient to intensive care unit or coronary care unit
7. Prompt consultation with cardiovascular surgeon

DIAGNOSTIC WORK-UP

1. Labs: CBC (leukocytosis as a stress reaction, low hemoglobin in ruptured dissection), BMP (elevated creatinine in dehydration or renal artery involvement), troponin, smooth muscle myosin heavy-chain assay ≥ 2.5 (sensitivity of 91%, specificity of 98%, and accuracy of 96%), urinalysis (hematuria due to renal artery involvement), and urine drug screen (cocaine).[1]
2. EKG to assess concomitant conditions, such as arrhythmias or ischemia.
3. Bedside chest X-ray, anteroposterior (AP) view, may demonstrate mediastinal widening $> 8\,cm$.[1]
4. In hemodynamically stable patients, CT angiography (CTA) of chest is the definitive test; two-dimensional (2D) or three-dimensional (3D) reconstructions improve detection rate.[1]
5. MRA (as accurate as CTA) in hemodynamically stable patients who have allergies to IV contrast.[1]
6. In hemodynamically unstable patients, bedside transthoracic echocardiogram (most useful in ascending aortic dissections) or bedside transesophageal echocardiogram (as accurate as CT/MRA for descending aortic dissection) are more appropriate tests.[1]

TREATMENT

1. Place arterial line for arterial blood pressure monitoring and central venous catheter; patient may need Swan-Ganz catheterization; patient may need Foley catheter for monitoring of urine output.
2. Decrease heart rate to target 60–80 beats/min[2,4] with:
   - Esmolol with loading dose of 500 µg/kg over 1 min, followed by 25 µg/kg/min; titrate to maximum 200 µg/kg/min[4]
   - Labetalol 10–20 mg IV bolus, followed by 1–2 mg/min to maximum of 300 mg over 24 h[4]
3. Decrease blood pressure to target 100–120 mmHg[2,4]; if blood pressure remains elevated despite β-blockers, consider:
   - Nitroglycerin 5 µg/min; increase by 5 µg/min every 3–5 min up to 20 µg/min[4]
4. Control pain with morphine 2–4 mg IV, every 2–4 h as needed.
5. Obtain cardiovascular surgery consultation for resection of the segment of the aorta with dissection and replacement with Dacron graft for:
   - Stanford type A (involving ascending aorta) aortic dissections.
   - Leaking/ruptured Stanford type B (involving descending aorta) aortic dissections
6. Uncomplicated descending aortic dissections are treated medically.

References

1. Mancini MC. *Aortic Dissection*. Emedicine.medscape.com. Updated: July 24, 2020.
2. Hiratzka LF, Beckman JA, Bersin RM, et al. 2010 Guidelines for the diagnosis and management of patients in thoracic aortic disease. American College of Cardiology Foundation and American Heart Association. *Circulation*. 2010;7:27–33.
3. Levy ZD, Zhou Q, Slesinger TL. Hypertensive crises. *Crit Care Emerg Med*. 2017;17:175–183.
4. Aronow WS. Treatment of hypertensive emergencies. *Ann Transl Med*. 2017;5(1):S5.

Acute Pericarditis

Presentation

Acute pericarditis is an inflammation of the pericardium due to various causes, including infection; medications (anticoagulants, hydralazine, isoniazid); radiation treatment; trauma to thorax; hypothyroidism; systemic diseases such as rheumatoid arthritis, ankylosing spondylitis, or sarcoidosis; and uremia or malignancy. Viral infections (adenovirus, coxsackie virus A and B, mumps, etc.) and idiopathic etiology are the most common causes. Acute pericarditis is diagnosed in 0.1% of patients hospitalized with chest pain.[1] Pericardial effusion that is refractory to treatment may lead to cardiac tamponade and hemodynamic compromise.

The most common symptom is chest pain that improves with the patient leaning forward.[2] Patient may describe chest pain as sharp and pleuritic. It is usually located in the retrosternal area. Pericardial rub may be present on cardiac auscultation. Symptoms of large pericardial effusion include hiccups, dysphagia, palpitation, presyncope, or syncope.

Causes for Rapid Response Activation

Persistently worsening chest pain, dyspnea, syncope.

Actions

INITIAL MEASURES

1. Continuous pulse oximetry
2. Supplemental oxygen to maintain $SpO_2 > 92\%$
3. Continuous cardiac monitoring

DIAGNOSTIC WORK-UP

1. Labs: CBC (leukocytosis), BMP, troponin (may be elevated in acute pericarditis), ESR (elevated), CRP (elevated), CK, TSH; if clinical presentation is suggestive of connective tissue disorder, order ANA and RF; consider HIV serology, QuantiFERON-TB assay, and blood cultures in patients with infectious etiology.
2. EKG may show widespread concave upward ST-segment elevation and PR-segment depression without T-wave inversions, with ST/T ratio > 0.25 in lead V6.[3]
3. Chest X-ray may demonstrate cardiomegaly, which, in the absence of known cardiac disease, indicates a pericardial effusion of at least 250 mL.[4]
4. Transthoracic echo to exclude pericardial effusion/tamponade.
5. If diagnosis is uncertain, cardiac CT scan or MRI with T2-weighted and late gadolinium enhancement will confirm pericardial inflammation and rule out myocarditis[5]; these studies will also allow measurement of pericardial thickness and will show loculated pericardial effusion.

TREATMENT

1. NSAIDs: aspirin 650–1000 mg orally four times a day, tapered over 4 weeks[6]; with a proton-pump inhibitor.
2. If pericarditis is refractory to NSAIDs, consider colchicine 0.6 mg twice daily for three months in patients weighing more than 154 lb (70 kg) or 0.6 mg once daily in patients weighing 154 lb or less[7]; colchicine reduces the risk of recurrence.
3. If acute pericarditis is caused by connective tissue disease or uremia, consider glucocorticoids, such as prednisone 1 mg/kg tapered over 2–3 weeks.[6]
4. Consult cardiovascular surgeon for pericardiocentesis in the following situations:
   - Cardiac tamponade
   - Hemodynamic compromise
   - Purulent, tuberculous, or neoplastic pericarditis suspected
   - Large (> 20 mm of echo-free space in diastole) pericardial effusion
   - Pericardial effusion that is refractory to treatment

References

1. Imazio M, Trinchero R. Current and future treatment for pericarditis. *Future Cardiol.* 2007;3(6):623–634.
2. Snyder MJ, et al. Acute pericarditis: diagnosis and management. *Am Fam Physician.* 2014;89(7):553–560.
3. Ginzton LE, Laks MM. The differential diagnosis of acute pericarditis from the normal variant: new electrocardiographic criteria. *Circulation.* 1982;65(5):1004–1009.
4. Lange RA, Hillis LD. Clinical practice. Acute pericarditis [published correction appears in *N Engl J Med.* 2005;352(11):1163]. *N Engl J Med.* 2004;351(21):2195–2202.
5. Bogaert J, Francone M. Cardiovascular magnetic resonance in pericardial diseases. *J Cardiovasc Magn Reson.* 2009;11:14.
6. Imazio M, Trinchero R. Triage and management of acute pericarditis. *Int J Cardiol.* 2007;118(3):286–294.
7. Imazio M, Brucato A, Cemin R, et al. ICAP Investigators. A randomized trial of colchicine for acute pericarditis. *N Engl J Med.* 2013;369(16):1522–1528.

Acute Cardiac Tamponade

Presentation

Cardiac tamponade is a compression of all cardiac chambers by accumulated pericardial fluid to the point of compromised systemic venous return to the right atrium, reduced chamber diastolic compliance, reduced ventricular filling, and decreased cardiac output.[1]

Symptoms include substernal chest pain that may radiate to the neck and jaw, accompanied by nausea, diaphoresis, and dyspnea. On physical exam patient may have tachypnea, sinus tachycardia, elevated jugular venous pressure, pulsus paradoxus, and pericardial friction rub.

Causes for Rapid Response Activation

Chest pain, dyspnea, signs of hypoperfusion, including hypotension, cold clammy extremities, decreased urine output, or worsening confusion.

Actions

INITIAL MEASURES

1. Continuous pulse oximetry
2. Supplemental oxygen to maintain $SpO_2 > 92\%$
3. Continuous cardiac monitoring
4. Bed rest with legs elevated to increase venous return
5. Transfer of patient to intensive care unit

DIAGNOSTIC WORK-UP

1. Labs: CBC (leukocytosis), BMP, troponin (may be elevated), ESR (elevated), CRP (elevated), CK, TSH; if clinical presentation is suggestive of connective tissue disorder, order ANA and RF; consider HIV serology and QuantiFERON-TB assay and blood cultures in patients with infectious etiology.
2. EKG may show sinus tachycardia, low QRS voltage ($< 0.5\,mV$) in limb leads, widespread concave upward ST-segment elevation, and PR-segment depression without T-wave inversions, or electrical alternans, which is an alteration of the QRS complex amplitude or axis between beats.[2]
3. Chest X-ray may demonstrate cardiomegaly, which, in the absence of known cardiac disease, indicates a pericardial effusion of at least $250\,mL$.[3]
4. Echocardiogram demonstrates late diastolic collapse of the right atrium and early diastolic collapse of right ventricle; persistence of right atrium collapse for more than one-third of the cardiac cycle is highly sensitive and specific for tamponade.

TREATMENT

1. Hypotensive patients will require volume expansion with saline, blood, or plasma.
2. Avoid positive mechanical ventilation, if possible, as it further reduces venous return and cardiac filling.[4]
3. In stable patients, treat underlying cause of the cardiac tamponade; in the meantime continue close hemodynamic monitoring and serial echocardiography.
4. Urgent percutaneous catheter pericardiocentesis in a cardiac catheterization lab is the definitive treatment for cardiac tamponade.[5]
5. For hemodynamically unstable patients, consult a cardiovascular surgeon for surgical removal of pericardial fluid through pericardial window.[5]

References

1. Spodick DH. Acute cardiac tamponade. *N Engl J Med.* 2003;349(7):684–690.
2. Bruch C, Schmermund A, Dagres N, et al. Changes in QRS voltage in cardiac tamponade and pericardial effusion: reversibility after pericardiocentesis and after anti-inflammatory drug treatment. *J Am Coll Cardiol.* 2001;38(1):219–226.
3. Lange RA, Hillis LD. Clinical practice. Acute pericarditis [published correction appears in *N Engl J Med.* 2005;352(11):1163]. *N Engl J Med.* 2004;351(21):2195–2202.
4. Little WC, Freeman GL. Pericardial disease. *Circulation.* 2006;113(12):1622–1632.
5. Yarlagadda C. *Cardiac Tamponade.* Emedicine.medscape.com. Updated: November 28, 2018.

CHAPTER 2

Respiratory Emergencies

Acute Asthma Exacerbation/Status Asthmaticus

Presentation

Asthma is characterized by airway inflammation that leads to episodic airway obstruction that is partially reversible.[1] Depending on the severity of symptoms, asthma exacerbation can be classified into mild, moderate, severe, and life-threatening.[2] Rapid response is usually activated for severe and life-threatening asthma exacerbations.

Severe asthma exacerbation is characterized by dyspnea at rest that interferes with conversation, peak expiratory flow (PEF) < 40% of predicted or personal best, and requires hospitalization. Life-threatening asthma exacerbation is characterized by an inability to speak due to dyspnea, accompanied by diaphoresis; PEF < 25% of predicted or personal best and requires transfer to ICU.[2]

Symptoms of asthma exacerbation include dyspnea, cough, wheezing, and chest tightness. On physical examination, patient will experience tachypnea, tachycardia, use of accessory muscles, intercostal retractions, decreased breath sounds, and inspiratory and expiratory wheezing.[2]

Causes for Rapid Response Activation

Worsening dyspnea, tachypnea, hypoxia, cyanosis, altered mental status.

Actions

INITIAL MEASURES

1. Continuous pulse oximetry
2. Supplemental oxygen to maintain SpO_2 > 90% or PaO_2 > 60–65 mmHg, transition to high flow oxygen when patient requires high flow rates
3. Continuous cardiac monitoring

DIAGNOSTIC WORK-UP

1. ABG in patients whose oxygen saturation is not restored to > 90% or whose FEV1 or PEF are ≤ 25% of predicted value, before and after initial treatment, allows assessment of asthma severity and response to treatment.[3]
2. Labs: CBC with differential (may demonstrate eosinophilia; eosinophils > 4% support the diagnosis of asthma[4]; patients with pneumonia might have leukocytosis) and BMP (assess electrolytes, renal function).

3. Administer EKG in patients age 50 and older and in patients with cardiac disease.
4. Chest X-ray will likely be normal or may show hyperinflation; it may be helpful to exclude other diseases and to assess complications such as lobar atelectasis, pneumonia, pneumothorax, and pneumomediastinum.[3]

TREATMENT

1. If the patient can tolerate it, measure PEF or forced expiratory volume in 1 second (FEV_1); an initial value should be obtained and repeated at 30–60 min after initial treatment to monitor treatment response; patients who are in respiratory extremis will benefit from PEF or FEV1 after they are stabilized.[2]
2. Maintain continuous albuterol 10–15 mg/ipratropium 1.5 mg nebulizer administration over 1 h.[3]
3. Administer prednisone 40–80 mg daily or methylprednisolone (Solumedrol) 125 mg IV, followed by 40–60 mg IV every 6–8 h; they have equivalent effects and should be administered until PEF reaches 70% of predicted or personal best.[3]
4. Consider magnesium sulfate 2 g IV over 20 min in patients with severe asthma exacerbation who are not improving after 1 h of intensive conventional treatment.[3]
5. In patients who are able to tolerate it and cooperate, consider a trial of BiPAP before intubation.
6. Start intubation and mechanical ventilation in patients with worsening respiratory status, such as:
   - Physical exhaustion
   - Decreasing level of consciousness
   - Respiratory muscle fatigue
   - Silent chest despite respiratory effort
   - Worsening hypoxia with SpO_2 < 90%
   - Worsening hypercapnia
   - Worsening acidosis with pH < 7.1
   - Hemodynamic instability
   - Comorbid conditions (MI, cardiac arrhythmias)[5]
7. Initial ventilator settings:
   - Mode of ventilation: assist control or pressure control.[5, 6]
   - Initial FiO_2: 100%; once the patient stabilizes, titrate it down to maintain SpO_2 at 90%–94%.
   - PEEP: 0–5 cmH₂O.
   - Tidal volume (VT) 6–8 mL/kg of predicted (ideal) body weight:
     - Male: PBW (kg) = 50 + 2.3(height(in)-60)
     - Female: PBW (kg) = 45.5 + 2.3(height(in)-60)
   - RR: 11–14 breaths per minute; titrate to maintain normal pH of 7.35–7.45.
   - Inspiratory to expiratory (I/E) ratio of 1:3.
   - Maintain plateau pressure (Pplat) ≤ 30 cmH₂O to avoid barotrauma.
   - Monitor clinical response, Pplat, and ABGs closely.[6]
8. Maintain intravascular volume in intubated patients with IV fluids such as normal saline, unless patient has pulmonary edema.

References

1. National Asthma Education and Prevention Program. Expert Panel Report 3 (EPR-3): Guidelines for the diagnosis and management of ASTHMA-summary report 2007. *J Allergy Clin Immunol.* 2007;120(5 Suppl):S94–138.
2. Pollart SM, Compton RM, Elward KS, et al. Management of acute asthma exacerbations. *Am Fam Physician.* 2011;84(1):40–47.

3. Camargo CA, et al. Managing asthma exacerbation in the emergency department. Summary of the National Asthma Education and Prevention Program Expert Panel Report 3. Guidelines for the management of asthma exacerbation. *Proc Am Thorac Soc.* 2009;6:357–366.
4. Morris MJ. *Asthma.* Emedicine.medscape.com. Updated November 20, 2020.
5. Hodder R, Lougheed MD, Fitz Gerald JM, et al. Management of acute asthma in adults in the emergency department: assisted ventilation. *CMAJ.* 2010;182(3):265–272.
6. Stather DR, Stewart TE. Clinical review: mechanical ventilation in severe asthma. *Crit Care.* 2005;9(6):581–587.

Chronic Obstructive Pulmonary Disease (COPD) Exacerbation

Presentation

Progression of COPD is characterized by thickening of the walls of the small airways and accumulation of inflammatory exudate in their lumens. COPD exacerbation is associated with a high mortality rate.

The most common precipitators of COPD exacerbation are acute respiratory infections caused by viruses such as human rhinovirus and bacteria (e.g., *Haemophilus influenzae, Moraxella catarrhalis, Streptococcus pneumoniae,* and *Pseudomonas aeruginosa*).[1] Environmental pollution and temperature changes are other contributing factors.[1]

COPD exacerbation is commonly manifested by progressively worsening cough, dyspnea, wheezing, increased sputum production, and purulent sputum.[1] Severe COPD exacerbation is characterized by respiration rate > 30 breaths per minute, use of accessory respiratory muscles, mental status changes, and $PaCO_2 > 50$ mmHg or increased from baseline.[1]

Causes for Rapid Response Activation

Worsening dyspnea at rest, tachypnea, significantly increased work of breathing, cyanosis, confusion, lethargy.

Actions

INITIAL MEASURES

1. Continuous pulse oximetry
2. Supplemental oxygen to maintain SpO_2 88%–92%[1] or $PaO_2 > 60$–65 mmHg, transition to high flow oxygen when patient requires high flow rates
3. Continuous cardiac monitoring

DIAGNOSTIC WORK-UP

1. Perform ABG to assess severity of hypoxia, hypercapnia, and respiratory acidosis; hypercapnia occurs when FEV1 decreases to $< 30\%$ of the predicted value.[2]
2. Labs: CBC (polycythemia; leukocytosis in patients with pneumonia), BMP (electrolyte abnormalities, renal function), magnesium, procalcitonin (elevated in bacterial or fungal infections).
3. Administer EKG in patients with concomitant cardiac disease, such as arrhythmia or ischemia.
4. Chest X-ray may demonstrate hyperinflated lungs, flat hemidiaphragms, increased anteroposterior diameter, bullous changes, and also show evidence of comorbid conditions such as congestive heart failure, pleural effusions, or pneumonia.[2]

TREATMENT

1. Administer albuterol/ipratropium (2.5 mg/0.5 mg)/3 mL NS nebulized.[3]
2. Administer oral corticosteroids:
   - 40 mg orally daily for 5 days[3]
3. Use IV corticosteroids in patients who are unable to tolerate oral corticosteroids or do not have gastrointestinal access for oral steroids[3]:
   - Methylprednisolone 60–120 mg IV daily for no longer than 5–7 days[3]
4. Antibiotics decrease short-term mortality, treatment failure, and sputum purulence and are indicated in the following situations:
   - Patient has three cardinal symptoms of COPD exacerbation: increased dyspnea, increased sputum production, and presence of purulent sputum.
   - Patient requires noninvasive or invasive ventilation.[4]
5. Administer antibiotics (nonpseudomonal coverage):
   - Ceftriaxone 1–2 g IV daily for 5–7 days
   - Moxifloxacin 400 mg PO/IV daily for 5–7 days[3]
6. Provide pseudomonal coverage:
   - Cefepime 1–2 g IV q 8–12 h for 5–7 days
   - Ceftazidime 1–2 g IV q 8 h for 5–7 days
   - Piperacillin-tazobactam 4.5 g IV q 6 h for 5–7 days
   - Levofloxacin 750 mg IV daily for 5–7 days[3]
7. Noninvasive positive pressure ventilation (NIPPV) reduces the need for intubation, mortality, length of ICU, and hospital stay.[4]
8. Indications for invasive PPV:

Major criteria (any one of the following):
   - Respiratory arrest
   - Loss of consciousness
   - Inadequate airway protection: aspiration, vomiting, inability to clear secretions
   - Psychomotor agitation (e.g., confusion or combativeness) requiring sedation
   - Hemodynamic instability with a systolic blood pressure < 70 mmHg
   - Heart rate < 50 beats/min with loss of alertness
   - Inability to tolerate NIPPV

Minor criteria (any two of the following):
   - Respiratory rate > 35 breath/min
   - Worsening acidemia or pH < 7.25
   - PaO_2 < 40 mm Hg, $PaCO_2$ > 60 mmHg, or PaO_2/FiO_2 < 200 mmHg despite oxygen therapy
   - Decreasing level of consciousness[5]

9. Initial ventilator settings:
   - Mode of ventilation: assist control.
   - Initial FiO_2: 100%; however, allow permissive hypercapnia and titrate it down to maintain SpO_2 at 88%–92%.
   - PEEP: no PEEP (due to auto-PEEP in COPD).
   - Tidal volume (VT) 6–8 mL/kg of predicted (ideal) body weight:
     - Male: PBW (kg) = 50 + 2.3(height(in)-60)
     - Female: PBW (kg) = 45.5 + 2.3(height(in)-60)
   - RR: 10–12 breaths per minute; titrate to maintain normal pH of 7.35–7.45.
   - Inspiratory to expiratory (I/E) ratio of 1:3.
   - Maintain plateau pressure (Pplat) ≤ 30 cmH$_2$O to avoid barotrauma.
   - Monitor clinical response, Pplat, and ABGs closely.[5]

References

1. *Global Initiative for Chronic Obstructive Lung Disease. Global Strategy for the Diagnosis, Management, and Prevention of Chronic Obstructive Pulmonary Disease*; 2018. Report http://goldcopd.org.
2. Mosenifar Z. *Chronic Obstructive Pulmonary Disease.* Emedicine.medscape.com. Updated: September 11, 2020.
3. Huntsberry A, Won K. Managing chronic and acute COPD exacerbations. *US Pharm.* 2018;43(7). HS-13-HS-16.
4. Wedzicha JA, Miravitlles M, Hurst JR, et al. Management of COPS exacerbations: a European Respiratory Society/American Thoracic Society guideline. *Eur Respir J.* 2017;49:1600791.
5. Mowery NT. Ventilator strategies for chronic obstructive pulmonary disease and acute respiratory distress syndrome. *Surg Clin N Am.* 2017;97:1381–1397.

Aspiration Pneumonitis

Presentation

Aspiration pneumonitis is a chemical inflammation of the lungs caused by inhalation of oropharyngeal contents or gastric acid into the lungs.[1] Impaired swallowing is the basic pathogenesis of the aspiration. Most aspiration events are unwitnessed.[2]

Predisposing conditions include altered consciousness resulting from drugs, general anesthesia, alcoholism, seizure, stroke, dementia, and neuromuscular disorders such as Parkinson's disease, myasthenia gravis, and multiple sclerosis. Patients with esophageal disorders such as achalasia, esophageal stricture, neoplasm, or diverticula are at high risk for aspiration.[1]

Gastric acid may cause bronchoconstriction, edema, atelectasis, and alveolar hemorrhage. Within a few minutes to 2 h of an aspiration event, patients with aspiration pneumonitis may develop hoarseness, dyspnea, audible wheezing, chest discomfort, cough with frothy sputum, fever, tachypnea, tachycardia, increased work of breathing, and hypoxia.[1]

Causes for Rapid Response Activation

Worsening dyspnea, tachypnea, labored breathing, hypoxia, cyanosis, altered mental status.

Actions

INITIAL MEASURES

1. Continuous pulse oximetry
2. Supplemental oxygen to maintain $SpO_2 > 92\%$ or $PaO_2 > 60-65$ mmHg, transition to high flow oxygen when patient requires high flow rates
3. Continuous cardiac monitoring
4. Adjust the patient's position to minimize further aspiration:
   - Semi-recumbent position
   - Elevate the head of the bed to 45° angle
   - Rotate patient's head laterally[2]

DIAGNOSTIC WORK-UP

1. ABG may demonstrate acute hypoxia and normal to low $PaCO_2$.[1]
2. Labs: CBC (leukocytosis will raise suspicion for pneumonia), magnesium, BMP (to assess electrolyte abnormalities and renal function), BNP (to assess fluid status), and procalcitonin (more likely to be elevated in aspiration pneumonia).
3. Chest X-ray may demonstrate unilateral or bilateral infiltrates or diffuse infiltrates that could resemble appearance of pulmonary edema, usually in dependent areas of lungs; patients may also develop pleural effusions.[1]
4. Consider CT scan of chest in patients with suspicion for empyema, necrosis within infiltrates, lung abscess, or cavitary lesions.
5. Order sputum, tracheal aspirate, or bronchoalveolar lavage cultures if infection is suspected.

TREATMENT

1. Administer humidified oxygen.
2. Suction the upper airway to remove aspirate.
3. Administer nebulized albuterol 2.5 mg/3 mL NS.
4. If aspiration of food or other foreign body is suspected, consult pulmonologist for bronchoscopy.[1]
5. If patient develops pleural effusion, consult interventional radiologist for thoracentesis[1] for diagnostic (exudate vs transudate, gram stain, cultures, LDH) and therapeutic (relief of dyspnea) purposes.
6. Intubate patients with acute respiratory distress syndrome or inability to protect the airway.[1,2]
7. In intubated patients, to prevent recurrent aspiration, insert a nasogastric tube to provide gastric decompression through either suction or gravity drainage.[2]
8. Consult interventional radiologist for placement of chest tube in patients with empyema.
9. When patient is stable, consult speech therapist for comprehensive swallowing evaluation and dietary recommendations (specialized texture diet, thickened liquids, chin tuck, etc.) and continue aspiration precautions (semirecumbent position, elevation of the head of the bed to 45° angle, etc.).
10. Antibiotics are not recommended for aspiration pneumonitis, but may be considered in the following cases:
    - Pneumonitis does not resolve within 48 h
    - Patients with small bowel obstruction
    - Patients taking antacids[1]
11. Antibiotic choices for community-acquired pathogens[1]:
    - Ceftriaxone 2 g IV daily[3] plus azithromycin 500 mg IV daily[4]
    - Levofloxacin 750 mg IV daily[5]
12. Antibiotic choices for hospital-acquired pathogens such as gram-negative bacteria, including *Pseudomonas aeruginosa*, *Klebsiella pneumoniae*, and MRSA[1]:
    - Piperacillin-tazobactam 4.5 g IV q 6 h[6] plus vancomycin 15 mg/kg IV q 12 h[7]
    - Imipenem/cilastatin 500 mg IV q 6 h[8] plus vancomycin 15 mg/kg IV q 12 h[7]

References

1. Gamache J. *Aspiration Pneumonitis and Pneumonia.* Emedicine.medscape.com. Updated: August 15, 2018.
2. Son YG, Shin J, Ryu HG. Pneumonitis and pneumonia after aspiration. *J Dent Anesth Pain Med.* 2017;17(1):1–12.
3. *Ceftriaxone.* Reference.medscape.com.
4. *Azithromycin.* Reference.medscape.com.
5. *Levofloxacin.* Reference.medscape.com.
6. *Piperacillin-Tazobactam.* Reference.medscape.com.
7. *Vancomycin.* Reference.medscape.com.
8. *Imipenem/Cilastatin.* Reference.medscape.com.

Life-Threatening Hemoptysis

Presentation

Hemoptysis is expectoration of blood from lung parenchyma or/and bronchial airways. Prior definitions of life-threatening hemoptysis ranged from 100 to 1000 mL of expectorated blood per 24 h.[1] However, the current definition of life-threatening hemoptysis reflects the rate of bleeding; airway obstruction and asphyxiation from blood; hemodynamic instability; abnormal ABG; known high-risk lesions, such as neoplasm, lung abscess, AVM; or lesions with pulmonary artery involvement.[2] Mortality rate from life-threatening hemoptysis can be as high as 80%, if untreated.[3]

Causes for Rapid Response Activation

Tachycardia, tachypnea, hypoxia, hypotension, aspiration of blood.

Actions

INITIAL MEASURES

1. Continuous pulse oximetry
2. Supplemental oxygen to maintain $SpO_2 > 92\%$ or $PaO_2 > 60–65$ mmHg, transition to high flow oxygen when patient requires high flow rates
3. Continuous cardiac monitoring
4. Consultation with pulmonologist and cardiovascular surgeon early in the process of rapid response

DIAGNOSTIC WORK-UP

1. Perform ABG to assess the severity of hypoxia.
2. Labs: CBC (hemoglobin and hematocrit, thrombocytopenia), coagulation studies (INR, PT, aPTT), BMP, blood typing and cross-match, D-dimer; after patient is stabilized, consider sputum culture (if infection is suspected), sputum AFB smear and culture (if TB is suspected), or sputum cytology (if neoplasm is suspected).
3. Chest X-ray may localize the source of bleeding and may show cavitary lesion, infiltrate, or mass.
4. Multiple detector CT angiography of chest in stable patients is superior to chest X-ray in identifying both the anatomic source and the cause of the hemorrhage.

TREATMENT

1. Once the bleeding side has been determined by chest X-ray, the patient should be placed in the lateral decubitus position with the affected lung down to prevent pooling of blood in the unaffected bronchial system.[4]
2. Start rapid volume resuscitation.

3. Blood product transfusion in hemodynamically stable patients includes[5]:
   - Packed red blood cells (RBC) if Hg < 7 g/dL; in cardiovascular patients if Hg < 8 g/dL
   - Fresh frozen plasma if INR > 1.6
   - Platelets if platelet count is < 50×10^9/L

4. Stop/reverse all anticoagulants with the following reversal options[6]:
   - IV heparin infusion or subcutaneous heparin-protamine 1 mg/100 U of heparin; maximum dose is 50 mg IV.
   - Subcutaneous enoxaparin (Lovenox)-protamine 0.5–1 mg/1 mg of enoxaparin; maximum dose is 50 mg IV.
   - Fondaparinux (Arixtra) (factor Xa inhibitor)-rFVIIa (NovoSeven) 90 µg/kg IV.
   - Warfarin-vitamin K 10 mg IV slowly over 30 min (onset of action in 2 h and is maximal at 24 h) and FFP 2–4 units or prothrombin complex concentrate (PCC) 25–50 IU/kg, activated PCC FEIBA (factor VIII inhibitor bypassing activity), or recombinant activated factor VIIa; target INR < 1.3–1.5.
   - Dabigatran (Pradaxa) (direct thrombin inhibitor)-idarucizumab (Praxbind); infuse 5 g dose IV as two consecutive 2.5 g infusions, a monoclonal antibody that directly targets dabigatran—treatment was approved by FDA in 2015; if idarucizumab is not available, consider 4-factor PCC (KCentra) 25–50 IU/kg; consider hemodialysis in patients with renal impairment.
   - Rivaroxaban (Xarelto) and apixaban (Eliquis) (factor Xa inhibitors)-andexanet (Andexxa) 400–800 mg IV depending on the dose and timing of the last dose; approved by FDA in 2018; if andexanet is not available, consider 4-factor PCC (KCentra) 25–50 IU/kg.
   - Activated charcoal 50–100 g via nasogastric tube may be administered if the ingestion is within 2–6 h for dabigatran, apixaban, and rivaroxaban.

5. For stable patients with no identifiable lesion on CXR, consult interventional radiologist for chest CT angiography and/or bronchial artery angiography with subsequent bronchial artery embolization (BAE).[7]

6. For unstable patients, consult pulmonology for immediate airway control with endotracheal intubation and flexible or rigid bronchoscopy.[8]

7. Intubate with large diameter ETT ≥ 8.5 mm inner diameter in order to pass therapeutic flexible bronchoscope for localization of hemorrhage and for placement of inflatable bronchial blocker, to evacuate blood clots from the airways, to direct instillation of ice-cold saline and/or epinephrine, or for use of thermoablative therapies such as electrocautery or argon plasma coagulation.[8]

8. Alternatively, selective intubation into the unaffected mainstem will allow isolation from the hemorrhage from the affected side.[8]

9. Once airway is stabilized and hemostasis is achieved, percutaneous bronchial artery embolization is the next step; an arteriogram will reveal bronchial arteries that normally originate from thoracic aorta at the level of T5 and T6; embolization agent or metallic coil will be placed at the site of bleeding, such as an aneurysm or arteriovenous malformation (AVM).[9]

10. After successful percutaneous bronchial artery embolization, definitive surgical treatment can be done by cardiothoracic surgeon as a scheduled intervention.

References

1. Bidwell JL, Pachner RW. Hemoptysis: diagnosis and management. *Am Fam Physician*. 2005;72(7):1253–1260.
2. Ibrahim WH. Massive haemoptysis: the definition should be revised. *Eur Respir J*. 2008;32(4):1131–1132.
3. Jean-Baptiste E. Clinical assessment and management of massive hemoptysis. *Crit Care Med*. 2000;28:1642–1647.

4. Earwood JS, Thompson TD. Hemoptysis: evaluation and management. *Am Fam Physician.* 2015;91(4):243–249.

5. Sharma S, Sharma P, Tyler LN. Transfusion of blood and blood products: indications and complications. *Am Fam Physician.* 2011;83(6):719–724.

6. Hanigan S, Barnes GD. *Managing Anticoagulant-Related Bleeding in Patients With Venous Thromboembolism.* American College of Cardiology; 2019. Acc.org.

7. Ketai LH, Mohammed TL, Kirsch J, et al, Expert Panel on Thoracic Imaging. ACR appropriateness criteria hemoptysis. *J Thorac Imaging.* 2014;29(3):W19–W22.

8. Sakr L, Dutau H. Massive hemoptysis: an update on the role of bronchoscopy in diagnosis and management. *Respiration.* 2010;80(1):38–58.

9. Davidson K, Shojaee S. Managing massive hemoptysis. *Chest.* 2020;157(1):77–88.

ARDS (Acute Respiratory Distress Syndrome)

Presentation

ARDS is a noncardiogenic pulmonary edema. Symptoms include dyspnea, tachypnea, and hypoxia that rapidly progress into acute respiratory failure. Onset of symptoms occurs within 1 week of a known pulmonary or extrapulmonary insult. Most cases of ARDS are associated with pneumonia with or without sepsis or with nonpulmonary sepsis.[1]

Older patients are at higher risk for ARDS. Other risk factors include aspiration, pulmonary contusion, burns, and transfusion-related acute lung injury, among others. Symptoms include fever, altered mental status, productive cough, pleuritic chest pain, decreased urine output, tachycardia, tachypnea, hypoxia, and hypotension.

Causes for Rapid Response Activation

Worsening dyspnea, increased work of breathing, tachypnea, tachycardia, profound hypoxia not responding to oxygen.

Actions

1. Continuous pulse oximetry
2. Supplemental oxygen to maintain $SpO_2 > 92\%$ or $PaO_2 > 60$–$65\,mmHg$; transition to high flow oxygen when patient requires high flow rates
3. Continuous cardiac monitoring
4. Suction secretions after positioning the jaw and tongue
5. Ventilation with bag-valve mask while preparing for NIPPV or invasive PPV
6. Consultation with pulmonologist or critical care specialist early in the process of rapid response

DIAGNOSTIC WORK-UP

1. Perform ABG to assess the severity of hypoxia and respiratory acidosis.
2. Labs: CBC (leukocytosis), BMP, lactic acid (elevated), CRP (elevated), procalcitonin (elevated in bacterial and fungal infections).
3. Chest X-ray may demonstrate bilateral pulmonary opacities.

TREATMENT

1. Promptly start invasive PPV—it is the only strategy to improve mortality.
2. Initial ventilator settings:
   - Mode of ventilation: volume assist control.
   - Initial FiO_2: 100%; once patient stabilizes, titrate it down to maintain SpO_2 at 88%–95% or PaO_2 55–80 mmHg.

- PEEP: 18–24 cm of H_2O; titrate down as you titrate down FiO_2.
- Tidal volume (VT) 6 mL/kg of predicted (ideal) body weight:
  - Male: PBW (kg) = 50 + 2.3(height(in)-60)
  - Female: PBW (kg) = 45.5 + 2.3(height(in)-60)
- RR: 14–22 breaths per minute.
- Inspiratory to expiratory (I/E) ratio of 1:1 to 1:3.
- Maintain plateau pressure (Pplat) $\leq 30\,cmH_2O$ to avoid barotrauma.[2]

3. Monitoring parameters:
   - Clinical response
   - Arterial pH of 7.3–7.45
   - SpO_2 of 88%–95%
   - PaO_2 of 55–80 mmHg
   - Plateau pressure $\leq 30\,cmH_2O$[2]
4. Prone position for 12–16 h a day[2]
5. The Surviving Sepsis Campaign guidelines recommend hydrocortisone 200 mg IV daily in patients with sepsis who are hemodynamically unstable despite fluid administration and vasopressor therapy.[3]
6. Use conservative fluid management therapy.
7. Patients with an anticipated ventilation requirement of at least 72 h should be started on enteral nutrition.[4]
8. May consider neuromuscular blocking agents to decrease patient-ventilator dyssynchrony and improve oxygenation when sedation alone is insufficient.
9. Consider early ECMO (extracorporeal membrane oxygenation) in refractory ARDS.
10. Once the patient starts to improve, initiate spontaneous breathing trials.
11. Provide mechanical and pharmacological VTE prophylaxis.

References

1. Rubenfeld GD, Caldwell E, Peabody E, et al. Incidence and outcomes of acute lung injury. *N Engl J Med.* 2005;353(16):1685–1693.
2. Saguil A, Fargo M. Acute respiratory distress syndrome: diagnosis and management. *Am Fam Physician.* 2020;101(12):730–738.
3. Rhodes A, Evans LE, Alhazzani W, et al. Surviving Sepsis Campaign: international guidelines for management of sepsis and septic shock: 2016. *Intensive Care Med.* 2017;43(3):304–377.
4. McClave SA, Taylor BE, Martindale RG, et al. Guidelines for the Provision and Assessment of Nutrition Support Therapy in the Adult Critically Ill Patient: Society of Critical Care Medicine (SCCM) and American Society for Parenteral and Enteral Nutrition (A.S.P.E.N.). *J Parenter Enter Nutr.* 2016;40(2):159–211.

Massive Pulmonary Embolism

Presentation

Massive pulmonary embolism is an acute PE with sustained systolic blood pressure < 90 mmHg for at least 15 min or requiring inotropic support, not due to a cause other than PE, such as arrhythmia, hypovolemia, sepsis or LV dysfunction, pulselessness, or persistent profound bradycardia with HR < 40 bpm with signs or symptoms of shock.[1] Symptoms of pulmonary embolism include dyspnea, chest pain, palpitations, dizziness, and syncope. On physical examination, patients may have tachycardia, tachypnea, or jugular vein distention.

Causes for Rapid Response Activation

Hypotension, syncope, worsening hypoxia.

Actions

INITIAL MEASURES

1. Continuous pulse oximetry
2. Supplemental oxygen to maintain SpO_2 > 92% or PaO_2 > 60–65 mmHg, transition to high flow oxygen when patient requires high flow rates
3. Continuous cardiac monitoring

DIAGNOSTIC WORK-UP

1. EKG may demonstrate sinus tachycardia, anterior precordial T-wave inversion, S1Q3T3, or precordial ST-segment elevation.[2]
2. STAT bedside transthoracic echocardiogram (TTE) (if no RV dilation, RV hypokinesis, septal shift, or tricuspid regurgitation—PE is unlikely).[1]
3. Confirm diagnosis with CT angio of thorax before reperfusion therapy even in patients with renal insufficiency unless patient is in severe hemodynamic instability.[1]
4. Avoid VQ scan (about 1 h of being out of ICU) or bilateral lower extremity Doppler ultrasound (if negative does not confirm absence of PE).[1]

TREATMENT

1. Avoid excessive IVF (worsens septal bowing into LV).
2. Administer vasopressor: norepinephrine is a vasopressor of choice:
   - Norepinephrine 8–12 µg/min IV infusion initially, with maintenance of 2–4 µg/min
3. Administer heparin drip[1]:

Initial dosage	Bolus of 80 units/kg, then 18 units/kg/h by infusion
APTT < 35 s (< 1.2 times control)	Bolus of 80 units/kg, then 4 units/kg/h by infusion
APTT = 35–45 s (1.2–1.5 times control)	Bolus of 40 units/kg, then 2 units/kg/h by infusion
APTT = 46–70 s (1.5–2.3 times control)	No change
APTT = 71–90 s (2.3–3.0 times control)	Decrease infusion rate by 2 units/kg/h
APTT > 90 s (> 3.0 times control)	Hold infusion for 1 h; then decrease infusion rate by 3 units/kg/h

4. For thrombolysis in patients with CTA-confirmed PE, hold heparin drip, administer alteplase (Activase) 100 mg IV over 2 h; thrombolysis will decrease mortality and recurrence of massive pulmonary embolism[3]; in submassive pulmonary embolism, thrombolysis does not reduce mortality, but it improves hemodynamics, reverses RV dilation, and prevents hemodynamic decompensation.[4]
5. After alteplase infusion is complete, check aPTT; if aPTT is < 80 s, restart heparin drip without bolus; if aPTT is ≥ 80 s, recheck aPTT in 4 h.
6. Consider catheter-directed thrombolysis/embolectomy or surgical embolectomy in patients with:
   - Contraindication to systemic thrombolytic therapy
   - Failed systemic thrombolytic therapy (persistent clinical instability and residual RV dysfunction on echo at 36 h)
   - Likelihood of dying before systemic thrombolytic therapy is complete
   - Relative contraindications to systemic thrombolytic therapy (half-dose thrombolytic can be used—alteplase 50 mg IV over 2 h—because it provides similar improvements in RV strain and pulmonary artery pressures)[5]
7. Once hemodynamic stability is achieved, transition the patient to direct oral anticoagulants:
   - Apixaban 10 mg po bid for 7 days, followed by 5 mg po bid[6]
   - Rivaroxaban 15 mg po bid for 21 days, followed by 20 mg po once a day[7]
8. Absolute contraindications to systemic thrombolytic therapy:
   - Acute or any prior intracranial hemorrhage
   - Arteriovenous malformation (AVM)
   - Malignant intracranial neoplasm
   - Ischemic stroke within last 3 months
   - Suspected aortic dissection
   - Coagulopathy (liver cirrhosis, ESRD, hematologic malignancy, vitamin K deficiency, antiphospholipid syndrome, INR > 1.7 or PT > 15 s, platelets < 100,000)
   - Neurosurgery (brain or spinal)
   - Serious head or facial trauma within last 3 months[8]
9. Relative contraindications:
   - Advanced age (older than 75 years)
   - Current anticoagulation with warfarin or new oral anticoagulants such as direct thrombin inhibitors (dabigatran or argatroban) or Factor Xa inhibitors (apixaban or rivaroxaban)
   - Pregnancy
   - Noncompressible vascular puncture
   - Traumatic or prolonged (> 10 min) CPR

- Recent internal bleeding such as GI or GU bleeding within the last 21 days
- Severe uncontrolled hypertension (BP > 180/110)
- Dementia
- Remote (> 3 months) ischemic stroke
- Recent major surgery
- Severe hyperglycemia (blood glucose > 400 mg/dL) or hypoglycemia (blood glucose < 50 mg/dL)
- Therapeutic doses of low-molecular-weight heparin

References

1. Wilbur J, Shian B. Deep venous thrombosis and pulmonary embolism: current therapy. *Am Fam Physician.* 2017;95(5):295–302.
2. Bernal AG, Fanola C, Bartos JA. *Management of Pulmonary Embolism.* American College of Cardiology; 2020. www.acc.org.
3. Wan S, Quinlan DJ, Agnelli G, Eikelboom JW. Thrombolysis compared with heparin for the initial treatment of pulmonary embolism: a meta-analysis of the randomized controlled trials. *Circulation.* 2004;110:744–749.
4. Meyer G, Vicaut E, Danays T, et al. Fibrinolysis for patients with intermediate-risk pulmonary embolism. *N Engl J Med.* 2014;370:1402–1411.
5. Wang C, Zhai Z, Yang Y, et al. Efficacy and safety of low dose recombinant tissue-type plasminogen activator for the treatment of acute pulmonary thromboembolism: a randomized, multicenter, controlled trial. *Chest.* 2010;137:254–262.
6. *Apixaban.* Reference.medscape.com.
7. *Rivaroxaban.* Reference.medscape.com.
8. Rivera-Bou WL. *What Are Absolute Contraindications for Use of Alteplase in Thrombolytic Therapy for Acute Ischemic Stroke (AIS)?* . Emedicine.medscape.com. Updated: December 31, 2017.

Severe Acute Atelectasis

Presentation

Atelectasis is a collapse affecting all or part of a lung. It is one of the most common radiographic abnormalities. Atelectasis can be obstructive (due to blocked airway such as tumor, foreign body, or mucus plug) and nonobstructive (due to pressure from outside the lung that prevents the lung from expansion, such as pleural effusion, pneumothorax, or large tumor).[1]

Atelectasis is a common postoperative complication. Conditions such as old age, smoking, dysphagia, obesity, sleep apnea, asthma, COPD, bronchiectasis, cystic fibrosis, and neuromuscular disorders increase the risk for atelectasis. Symptoms may include productive cough, wheezing, difficulty breathing, shallow breathing, tachypnea, tachycardia, and hypoxia.[1]

Causes for Rapid Response Activation

Sudden onset of worsening dyspnea, cyanosis, hypoxia.

Actions

INITIAL MEASURES

1. Continuous pulse oximetry
2. Supplemental oxygen to maintain $SpO_2 > 92\%$ or $PaO_2 > 60-65\,mmHg$, transition to high flow oxygen when patient requires high flow rates
3. Continuous cardiac monitoring
4. Place the patient in a position that leaves the unaffected side dependent to promote increased drainage of the affected area

DIAGNOSTIC WORK-UP

1. ABG to assess severity of hypoxia.
2. Labs: CBC (leukocytosis), BMP (concomitant electrolyte abnormalities, renal failure), procalcitonin (elevated in superimposed fungal or bacterial infections).
3. Sputum and blood cultures if superimposed infection is suspected.
4. Chest X-ray may demonstrate opacification and volume loss of the collapsed lobe or of the entire collapsed lung; indirect signs of atelectasis include mediastinal shift toward the side of collapse, elevation of ipsilateral diaphragm, and elevation of ipsilateral hilum.[1]

TREATMENT

1. As narcotics suppress coughing, use them sparingly.
2. Avoid antitussive medications, as they reduce the cough reflex and may contribute to further atelectasis.
3. Use techniques such as coughing, deep breathing, early ambulation, and forced expiration; incentive spirometry; acapella; suctioning; chest physiotherapy, including postural drainage; and chest wall percussion and vibration.

4. Use nebulized bronchodilators:
   - Albuterol 2.5 mg/3 mL NS nebulized[2]
5. Administer nebulized dornase alpha (DNase or Pulmozyme) 2.5 mg nebulizer once or twice daily.[3]
6. Start CPAP to improve oxygenation and reexpansion of the collapsed lung.
7. If these efforts are not successful within 24 h, are contraindicated, or are poorly tolerated, consult pulmonologist for flexible fiberoptic bronchoscopy, which will allow removal of mucus plug.
8. Bronchoscopy is required for the diagnosis of an endobronchial lesion, by washing, brushing, and biopsy of obstructing mass.
9. Antibiotics are not recommended for treatment of atelectasis without evidence of superimposed bacterial infection.
10. The antibiotic should target the specific pathogens isolated from sputum samples or bronchial secretions.[1]
    - Antibiotic choices for community-acquired pathogens:
      - Ceftriaxone 2 g IV daily[4] plus azithromycin 500 mg IV daily[5]
      - Cefuroxime 750 mg IV q 8 h[6]
      - Levofloxacin 750 mg IV daily[7]
    - Antibiotic choices for hospital-acquired pathogens such as gram-negative bacteria, including *Pseudomonas aeruginosa, Klebsiella pneumoniae,* and MRSA:
      - Piperacillin-tazobactam 4.5 g IV q 6 h[8] plus vancomycin 15 mg/kg IV q 12 h[9]
      - Imipenem/cilastatin 500 mg IV q 6 h[10] plus vancomycin 15 mg/kg IV q 12 h[9]
11. In patients with severe acute respiratory distress and hypoxia, proceed with intubation and mechanical ventilation.

References

1. Madappa T. *Atelectasis Treatment and Management.* December 6, 2018 Emedicine.medscape.com.
2. *Albuterol.* Reference.medscape.com.
3. Hendriks T, et al. DNase and atelectasis in non-cystic fibrosis pediatric patients. *Crit Care.* 2005; 9(4):R351–R356.
4. *Ceftriaxone.* Reference.medscape.com.
5. *Azithromycin.* Reference.medscape.com.
6. *Cefuroxime.* Reference.medscape.com.
7. *Levofloxacin.* Reference.medscape.com.
8. *Piperacillin-Tazobactam.* Reference.medscape.com.
9. *Vancomycin.* Reference.medscape.com.
10. *Imipenem/Cilastatin.* Reference.medscape.com.

Spontaneous Pneumothorax

Presentation

Pneumothorax is a presence of air in the pleural cavity that can impair oxygenation and ventilation. Spontaneous pneumothorax occurs when asymptomatic blebs or bullae rupture. This is accompanied by acute onset of stabbing pleuritic chest pain that may radiate to shoulder, shortness of breath, tachycardia, and tachypnea. Spontaneous pneumothorax can be primary and secondary.[1]

Primary pneumothorax occurs in patients without underlying lung disease in the absence of an inciting event. These patients have pleural blebs or bullae that can be detected by a CT scan of the chest. Usually, these patients smoke and are 18–40 years old, thin, and tall.[1] This type of pneumothorax usually occurs in patients with genetic disorders such as Marfan syndrome or homocystinuria.

Secondary spontaneous pneumothorax may occur in patients with parenchymal lung disease when air enters the pleural cavity from the damaged alveoli. Chronic pulmonary conditions such as asthma, COPD, cystic fibrosis, sarcoidosis, bronchogenic carcinoma, idiopathic pulmonary fibrosis, or pulmonary TB can cause secondary spontaneous pneumothorax.[1]

Causes for Rapid Response Activation

Progressively worsening chest pain, dyspnea, tachypnea, tachycardia, hypoxia.

Actions

INITIAL MEASURES

1. Continuous pulse oximetry
2. Supplemental oxygen to maintain $SpO_2 > 92\%$ or $PaO_2 > 60$–65 mmHg, transition to high flow oxygen when patient requires high flow rates
3. Continuous cardiac monitoring

DIAGNOSTIC WORK-UP

1. ABG—treatment should not be delayed while awaiting the results—may be useful to evaluate the severity of hypoxia, hypercarbia, and respiratory acidosis.[1]
2. Chest X-ray—not for confirmation of the diagnosis, but when patient is stable to assess extent of pneumothorax and potential causes.[1]
3. Bedside ultrasonography for hemodynamically unstable patients.[1]

TREATMENT

1. Unstable patients should be treated with needle aspiration: place a large-bore 14- to 16-gauge, 4.5-cm-long angiocatheter superior to the rib, in the second intercostal space in the midclavicular line, as a temporary measure.[2]
2. In stable patients with primary spontaneous pneumothorax:

- If pneumothorax is < 15% and patient is asymptomatic, treatment of choice is observation and administration of 100% oxygen to promote resolution.
- If pneumothorax is < 15% and the patient is symptomatic, needle aspiration is treatment of choice.
- If pneumothorax is > 15%, treatment of choice is aspiration with pigtail catheter left to low suction or water seal.[1]

3. In stable secondary spontaneous pneumothorax, treatment of choice is tube thoracostomy.[1]
4. If patient has experienced recurrent pneumothorax or if the lung remains unexpanded after 5 days with a chest tube in place, consult cardiovascular surgeon to consider:
   - Video-assisted thoracoscopic surgery (VATS)
   - Electrocautery: pleurodesis or sclerotherapy
   - Laser treatment
   - Resection of blebs or pleura
   - Open thoracotomy[1]

References

1. Daley BJ, Bhimji S, Bascom R, Benninghoff MG, Alam S. *Pneumothorax Treatment and Management.* Emedicine.medscape.com. Updated: April 28, 2020.
2. McKnight CL, Burns B. *Pneumothorax.* StatPearls Publishing. Ncbi.nim.nih.gov. Last Update: November 16, 2020.

Tension Pneumothorax

Presentation

Tension pneumothorax is characterized by injured tissue which forms a one-way valve allowing air inflow in pleural space with inhalation and prohibiting an air outflow. Air is trapped in the pleural cavity under positive pressure. Significant pneumothorax can cause mediastinal shift leading to impaired venous return and hemodynamic compromise. Symptoms include chest pain, dyspnea, diaphoresis, altered mental status, hypoxia, hypotension, jugular venous distention, cyanosis, asymmetric lung expansion, tachycardia (when HR > 135, tension pneumothorax is likely), followed by cardiac arrest and death.[1]

In the hospital, tension pneumothorax may happen in mechanically ventilated patients. Patients at risk are those with tidal volume greater than 12 mL/kg, a peak airway pressure greater than 60 cmH$_2$O, or a positive end-expiratory pressure greater than 15 cmH$_2$O.[1] Tension pneumothorax in mechanically ventilated patients may manifest with progressive difficulty with ventilation, sudden fall in SpO$_2$, followed by hypotension (over a few minutes), and subcutaneous emphysema.[2] Other signs include tachycardia, decreased breath sounds, hyperresonance, and tracheal deviation.[2] Patients on pressure-controlled ventilation may have a sudden drop in tidal volume.[1]

Patients who already have chest tube may still develop tension pneumothorax, as chest tubes may become plugged or malpositioned.[1]

Other causes of iatrogenic tension pneumothorax in the hospital setting include inadvertent intubation of right mainstem bronchus, transthoracic needle aspiration of pulmonary nodule (most common postprocedural cause, 32%–37% of cases), therapeutic thoracentesis, subclavian or internal jugular central vein placement, CPR, or nasogastric feeding tube placement.[1]

Causes for Rapid Response Activation

Chest pain, dyspnea, altered mental status, hypoxia, hypotension, cyanosis, tachycardia.

Actions

INITIAL MEASURES

1. Continuous pulse oximetry
2. Supplemental oxygen to maintain SpO$_2$ > 92% or PaO$_2$ > 60–65 mmHg, transition to high flow oxygen when patient requires high flow rates
3. Continuous cardiac monitoring

DIAGNOSTIC WORK-UP

1. ABG—treatment should not be delayed while awaiting the results—may be useful to evaluate the severity of hypoxia, hypercarbia, and respiratory acidosis.[1]
2. Chest X-ray—not for confirmation of the diagnosis, but when patient is stable to assess extent of pneumothorax and potential causes[1]; chest X-ray will show ipsilateral hyperexpansion and ipsilateral flattening of the heart border with contralateral mediastinal deviation.[2]
3. Bedside ultrasonography for hemodynamically unstable patients.[1]

TREATMENT

1. Use emergent needle decompression—for example, a 14G (4.5 cm) intravenous cannula can be inserted in the second intercostal space in the midclavicular line, in the cephalad border of the rib to avoid intercostal vessels in the lower edge of the rib; emergent needle decompression is done to gain time before a larger chest tube (tube thoracostomy) can be inserted.[1]
2. In patients with chest wall > 5 cm, the trocar (7 cm) may be considered.[2]
3. The use of the fourth or fifth intercostal space in the mid-axillary line may be safer and has been recommended by the advance trauma life support (ATLS) training program as it contains less fat and allows large muscles to be avoided; however, this access can potentially increase the risk of lung injury in the supine patient, as gas collects at the highest point, and adhesions are most likely in more dependent parts of the lung.[2]
4. If the patient has had recurrent pneumothorax or if the lung remains unexpanded after 5 days with a chest tube in place, consult cardiovascular surgeon to consider:
   - Video-assisted thoracoscopic surgery (VATS)
   - Electrocautery: pleurodesis or sclerotherapy
   - Laser treatment
   - Resection of blebs or pleura
   - Open thoracotomy[1]

References

1. Daley BJ, Bhimji S, Bascom R, Benninghoff MG, Alam S. *Pneumothorax Treatment and Management*. April 28, 2020. Emedicine.medscape.com.
2. Leigh-Smith S, Harris T. Tension pneumothorax – time for a re-think? *Emerg Med J.* 2005;22:8–16.

Acute Hypercapnic Respiratory Failure Due to Oversedation

Presentation

Opioids have the potential to cause significant respiratory depression; however, opioid treatment of moderate-to-severe pain is generally safe with $\leq 0.5\%$ of the events related to respiratory depression.[1] Patients who are most commonly at high risk for this condition are those with acute exacerbation of COPD who are also taking opioids for chronic pain.[2]

The risk for opioid-induced respiratory depression is common in the immediate postoperative recovery period. Drugs that decrease respiratory effort include barbiturates, benzodiazepines, antihistamines, and gabapentinoids such as gabapentin and pregabalin.

Besides COPD and asthma, neuromuscular disorders such as myasthenia gravis, chest wall disorders such as severe kyphoscoliosis, and central hypoventilation and obesity hypoventilation syndromes may increase risk for acute hypercapnic respiratory failure.

Symptoms include dyspnea, wheezing, and tachypnea. Despite treatment of COPD exacerbation with nebulized bronchodilators, steroids and BiPAP, and correction of hypercapnia, the patient may develop worsening altered mental status such as drowsiness and eventually unresponsiveness. On examination, the patient may have pinpoint pupils and bradypnea.

The Centers for Medicare and Medicaid Services (CMS) updated their recommendations in 2014 for hospital administration of opioids. A CMS-supported expert panel recommended a monitoring frequency of q 2.5 h for the first 24 h postoperatively and q 4.5 h afterward for an opioid administration.[3]

Causes for Rapid Response Activation

Worsening altered mental status, such as somnolence and bradypnea.

Actions

INITIAL MEASURES

1. Continuous pulse oximetry
2. Waveform capnography to monitor respiratory rate and $EtCO_2$
3. Supplemental oxygen to maintain $SpO_2 > 92\%$ (88%–92% in COPD patients) or $PaO_2 > 60$–65 mmHg, transition to high flow oxygen when patient requires high flow rates
4. Consideration of heated humidification, if respiratory secretions are thick and tenacious
5. Continuous cardiac monitoring
6. Frequent Glasgow Coma Scale (GCS) for monitoring of mental status
7. Consideration of other underlying cardiopulmonary conditions that could be contributing to worsening respiratory status

DIAGNOSTIC WORK-UP

1. ABG will likely demonstrate respiratory acidosis, elevated $PaCO_2$, and decreased PaO_2.
2. Labs: CBC (leukocytosis), BMP, BNP, and procalcitonin.
3. Order chest X-ray to assess any concomitant underlying cardiopulmonary condition.

TREATMENT

1. Administer naloxone 20–100 µg IV every 2 min as needed; onset of action is usually < 2 min; titrate to respiratory rate.[4]
2. Naloxone IV infusion 20–50 µg/h may be required.[4]
3. Monitor naloxone administration for side effects such as severe pain, stress, agitation, pulmonary edema, arrhythmias, and hypertension.
4. Early orotracheal intubation and invasive mechanical ventilation for patients unable to maintain patent airway and with severe respiratory depression.

References

1. Dahan A, Aarts L, Smith TW. Incidence, reversal, and prevention of opioid-induced respiratory depression. *Anesthesiology.* 2010;112:226–238.
2. Steynor M, MacDuff A. Always consider the possibility of opioid induced respiratory depression in patients presenting with hypercapnic respiratory failure who fail to improve as expected with appropriate therapy. *Case Rep Crit Care.* 2015;2015. Article ID 562319, 3 pp.
3. *Requirements for Hospital Medication Administration, Particularly Intravenous (IV) Medications and Post-Operative Care of Patients Receiving IV Opioids.* March 14, 2014 https://www.cms.gov/Medicare/Provider-Enrollment-and-Cert-Letter-14-15.pdf.
4. Boland J, Boland E, Brooks D. Importance of correct diagnosis of opioid-induced respiratory depression in adult cancer patients and titration of naloxone. *Clin Med.* 2013;13(2):149–151.

Acute Partial Upper Airway Obstruction

Presentation

In a hospital setting, patients may aspirate foreign bodies such as pills, food (peas, nuts), or dental appliances. Patients with dementia, stroke, parkinsonism, seizures, or mental delay have higher risk for foreign body aspiration. In adults, foreign bodies tend to become lodged in the right main bronchus due to its more vertical course and larger diameter.[1]

Symptoms may include coughing, gagging, chocking, dysphonia, dysphagia, odynophagia, stridor, and wheezing; however, patients are able to *vocalize and maintain their airway*.[1] On physical examination, patients may have wheezing and decreased breath sounds on the side of the foreign body. Lodging of the foreign object may lead to cessation of these symptoms.

Foreign body aspiration can be misdiagnosed as asthma or COPD exacerbation, especially in elderly patients with dementia or altered mental status. If untreated, retained foreign bodies may lead to complications, such as recurrent pneumonia, bronchiectasis, pneumothorax, pneumomediastinum, and lung abscess.

Causes for Rapid Response Activation

Worsening stridor, wheezing, dyspnea, tachypnea, hypoxia.

Actions

INITIAL MEASURES

1. Continuous pulse oximetry
2. Supplemental oxygen to maintain $SpO_2 > 92\%$ or $PaO_2 > 60–65$ mmHg, transition to high flow oxygen when patient requires high flow rates
3. Continuous cardiac monitoring

DIAGNOSTIC WORK-UP

1. ABG will assess the severity of hypoxia.
2. Order standard posteroanterior inspiratory and lateral chest radiography to look for unilateral hyperinflation and lobar or segmental atelectasis; a chest X-ray will demonstrate only radiopaque foreign bodies, such as teeth and dental appliances, in less than 25% of patients[2]; most foreign bodies are radiolucent, that is, not visible (e.g., pills, food, plastic foreign objects)[3]; patients with foreign body aspiration may have a normal chest X-ray.
3. If there is a reduction or cessation of symptoms, the foreign body has likely lodged in a mainstem or lower bronchi; in this case, perform a CT scan of the thorax, as the majority of foreign bodies are radiolucent, which is more sensitive for foreign body identification.

TREATMENT

1. NPO.
2. Have the patient assume position of comfort.
3. Avoid Heimlich maneuver, as this can convert partial obstruction to complete obstruction.[4]
4. In patients with stridor, administer racemic epinephrine nebulizer to decrease edema and bronchospasm:
   - Racemic epinephrine 0.5 mL of 2.25% solution diluted in 3 mL NS via jet nebulizer q 3–4 h PRN[5]
5. Pulmonology consultation for flexible bronchoscopy in OR, which has a 90% success rate for retrieval and allows a more comprehensive airway survey; grasping devices include forceps, baskets, or snares; rigid bronchoscopy is more optimal choice for patients with hemoptysis as the operator may use its barrel to mechanically tamponade the site of bleeding, and it also allows passage of the suction catheter; rigid bronchoscopy is preferred in patients with stridor/asphyxia.[4]
6. Postoperatively, chest physiotherapy may be used for patients with secretions.

References

1. Heim SW, Maughan KL. Foreign bodies in the ear, nose, and throat. *Am Fam Physician.* 2007; 76(8):1185–1189.
2. Hewlett JC, et al. Foreign body aspiration in adult airways: therapeutic approach. *J Thorac Dis.* 2017; 9(9):3398–3409.
3. Bloom DC, et al. Plastic laryngeal foreign bodies in children: a diagnostic challenge. *Int J Pediatr Otorhinolaryngol.* 2005;69:657–662.
4. Murray AD, Talavera F, Meyers AD. Foreign Bodies of the Airway. Emedicine.medscape.com. Updated: May 07, 2019.
5. *Racemic epinephrine.* Reference.Medscape.com.

Acute Complete Upper Airway Obstruction

Presentation

A large foreign body may lodge in larynx or trachea and cause complete obstruction due to the size of the foreign object and edema. Patients with acute complete upper airway obstruction are *aphonic and are unable to breathe*, as the foreign body completely obstructs the larynx or trachea. These patients can also have wheezing. [1,2]

Causes for Rapid Response Activation

Respiratory arrest.

Actions

INITIAL MEASURES

1. Continuous pulse oximetry
2. Supplemental oxygen to maintain $SpO_2 > 92\%$ or $PaO_2 > 60–65\,mmHg$, transition to high flow oxygen when patient requires high flow rates
3. Continuous cardiac monitoring

TREATMENT

1. NPO.
2. Heimlich maneuver if patient is conscious. [3]
3. If obstruction is relieved, place the patient in recovery position or position of comfort. [3]
4. If patient becomes unconscious, lower patient to the ground and start CPR (no pulse check) until equipment is ready for intubation. [3]
5. Avoid bag-mask ventilation as it can cause supraglottic foreign body to move below the vocal cords, making removal difficult. [3]
6. Perform direct laryngoscopy and attempt removal of foreign body using Magill forceps, if you can see the foreign body. [3]
7. If unable to remove the foreign body, intubate the right or left main stem bronchus, pushing the foreign body to enter the bronchus; then retract the tube to a proper depth, reinflate the cuff, and start invasive PPV. [3]
8. One lung ventilation must be done carefully with low respiratory rates and low tidal volumes to avoid pneumothorax. [3]
9. Pulmonology consultation for flexible bronchoscopy in OR, which has a 90% success rate for retrieval and allows a more comprehensive airway survey; grasping devices include forceps, baskets, or snares; rigid bronchoscopy is more optimal choice for patients with

hemoptysis as the operator may use its barrel to mechanically tamponade the site of bleeding, and it also allows passage of the suction catheter; rigid bronchoscopy is preferred in patients with stridor or asphyxia.[4]

10. Postoperatively, chest physiotherapy may be used for patients with secretions.

References

1. Hewlett JC, et al. Foreign body aspiration in adult airways: therapeutic approach. *J Thorac Dis.* 2017;9(9):3398–3409.
2. Heim ST, Maughan KL. Foreign bodies in the ear, nose and throat. *Am Fam Physician.* 2007;76(8):1185–1189.
3. Walls R. *Manual of Emergency Airway Management.* 4th ed; 2012:418–423. 8(40).
4. Murray AD, Talavera F, Meyers AD. Foreign Bodies of the Airway. Emedicine.medscape.com. Updated: May 07, 2019.

Idiopathic Pulmonary Fibrosis Exacerbation

Presentation

Idiopathic pulmonary fibrosis is a progressively worsening fibrotic lung disease of unknown etiology. Usually the disease occurs in adults in their 50s and 60s. Prognosis is poor with the median survival rate of 2–3 years from the time of diagnosis.[1] Mortality rate in acute exacerbation of idiopathic pulmonary fibrosis can be as high as 85%.[2]

The main symptoms of acute exacerbation are progressively worsening dyspnea and cough. Other symptoms could be flu-like symptoms such as fatigue, low-grade fevers, arthralgias, and myalgias. On physical examination, patients are tachypneic, have labored breathing, and have bibasilar crackles on lung auscultation.[2]

Causes for Rapid Response Activation

Persistently worsening dyspnea, labored breathing, hypoxia.

Actions

INITIAL MEASURES

1. Continuous pulse oximetry
2. Supplemental oxygen to maintain $SpO_2 > 92\%$ or $PaO_2 > 60$–$65\,mmHg$, transition to high flow oxygen when patient requires high flow rates
3. Continuous cardiac monitoring

DIAGNOSTIC WORK-UP

1. ABG may demonstrate decrease in the PaO_2 of $10\,mmHg$ or more from baseline.
2. Labs: CBC with differential cell count (may show leukocytosis even in the absence of infection), CRP (elevated), ESR (elevated), procalcitonin (elevated in bacterial and fungal infection), BNP (to assess fluid status), and D-dimer (patients with idiopathic pulmonary fibrosis are at high risk for venous thromboembolism).
3. If infection is suspected, order blood cultures, sputum cultures, *Streptococcus pneumoniae* and *Legionella* urinary antigen tests, and rapid influenza antigen test in appropriate season.
4. Chest X-ray will show peripheral reticular opacities mostly involving lung bases and also may show concomitant conditions such as pneumonia, pneumothorax, or pulmonary edema.[3]
5. High resolution CT scan (with or without PE protocol) will show new bilateral ground-glass consolidation superimposed on usual background peripheral and basal reticular opacities, honeycombing, and traction bronchiectasis.[3]

TREATMENT

1. High dose corticosteroids, for example, methylprednisolone 500–1000 mg IV daily for 3 days followed by a prolonged prednisone taper over the course of weeks to months (not evidence-based, consensus guideline, no decrease in mortality)[4,5]; only 10%–15% of patients will improve with corticosteroids; however, approximately 26% of patients will develop side effects due to the corticosteroids.[6]
2. Immunosuppressive medications such as cyclophosphamide 500 mg/m^2 IV bolus every 3 weeks[4,5] combined with corticosteroids improved 3-year survival rate.[6]
3. Broad spectrum IV antibiotics in patients with evidence of superimposed infection or elevated procalcitonin; antibiotics can be deescalated once the results of blood or sputum cultures are available; the usual course of treatment is 7 days.[5]
4. Noninvasive mechanical ventilation.
5. Invasive mechanical ventilation is of no benefit, except in younger patients, patients with fewer comorbidities, shorter time from diagnosis (accounting for the fact that average survival is 2–3 years), and those who will receive lung transplantation within the next few days.[5]
6. Neuromuscular blockade is acceptable to reduce lung stress and strain and patient-ventilator asynchrony.[7]
7. Initial ventilator settings:
   - Mode of ventilation: pressure- or volume-controlled.
   - Initial FiO$_2$: 100%; once the patient stabilizes, titrate it down to maintain SpO$_2$ at 90%–95% or PaO$_2$ 55–80 mmHg.
   - Low-moderate PEEP: 4–6 cm of H$_2$O; titrate down as you titrate down FiO$_2$.
   - Tidal volume (VT) 6 mL/kg of predicted (ideal) body weight:
     - Male: PBW (kg) = 50 + 2.3(height(in)-60)
     - Female: PBW (kg) = 45.5 + 2.3(height(in)-60)
   - Higher RR: 18–22 breaths per minute, to allow permissive hypercapnia.
   - Inspiratory to expiratory (I/E) ratio of 1:2.
   - Maintain plateau pressure (Pplat) $\leq$ 30 cmH$_2$O to avoid barotrauma.[7]
8. Prone position 16 h/day.[7]
9. Consult pulmonologist for flexible bronchoscopy with bronchoalveolar lavage (BAL) to exclude infectious etiology or malignancy; BAL samples should be submitted for stains and cultures for bacteria, mycobacteria, and fungi; run viral PCR panel.
10. Extracorporeal membrane oxygenation (ECMO) can be used as a bridge to lung transplantation, which is the only treatment associated with prolonged survival.

References

1. Schwartz DA, Helmers RA, Galvin JR, et al. Determinants of survival in idiopathic pulmonary fibrosis. *Am J Respir Crit Care Med.* 1994;149:450–454.
2. Song JW, Hong SB, Lim CM, et al. Acute exacerbation of idiopathic pulmonary fibrosis: incidence, risk factors and outcome. *Eur Respir J.* 2011;37:356–363.
3. Summerhill EM. *Interstitial Pulmonary Fibrosis.* Emedicine.medscape.com. Updated: September 15, 2020.
4. Raghu G, Collard HR, Egan JJ, et al. An official ATS/ERS/JRS/ALAT statement: idiopathic pulmonary fibrosis: evidence-based guidelines for diagnosis and management. *Am J Respir Crit Care Med.* 2011;183(6):788–824.
5. Juarez MM, Chan AL, Norris AG. Acute exacerbation of idiopathic pulmonary fibrosis – a review of current and novel pharmacotherapies. *J Thorac Dis.* 2015;7(3):499–519.
6. Kirchner JT. Diagnosis and management of idiopathic pulmonary fibrosis. *Am Fam Physician.* 1998;57(10):2527–2528.
7. Marchioni A, Tonelli R, Ball L, et al. Acute exacerbation of idiopathic pulmonary fibrosis: lessons learned from acute respiratory distress syndrome? *Crit Care.* 2018;22:80.

Acute Pulmonary Arterial Hypertension

Presentation

Pulmonary hypertension is characterized by a mean pulmonary arterial pressure of ≥ 25 mmHg at rest during right-heart catheterization.[1] Etiologies include idiopathic, inheritable, HIV, connective tissue disease, congenital heart disease, schistosomiasis, drugs, and toxins.

Acute pulmonary hypertension is acute right-sided heart failure in chronic pulmonary arterial hypertension resulting from reduced right ventricular filling and reduced right ventricular output. It can be precipitated by SVT (supraventricular tachycardia), infection/sepsis, pulmonary embolism, and vascular or cardiothoracic surgery. Prognosis is very poor.

Symptoms include progressively worsening fatigue, shortness of breath, chest pain, syncope, hemoptysis, lower extremity edema, ascites, anasarca, and palpitations. On physical examination, patients may have elevated jugular venous pressure, tachycardia, arrhythmias, ascites, and lower extremity edema.

Causes for Rapid Response Activation

Worsening dyspnea, chest pain, syncope, cyanosis, tachycardia.

Actions

INITIAL MEASURES

1. Continuous pulse oximetry
2. Supplemental oxygen to maintain $SpO_2 > 92\%$ or $PaO_2 > 60\text{--}65$ mmHg, transition to high flow oxygen when patient requires high flow rates
3. Continuous cardiac monitoring

DIAGNOSTIC WORK-UP

1. Labs: CBC (leukocytosis if infection is present), procalcitonin (elevated in bacterial and fungal infection), BNP (reduction of serial BNP is associated with good response to therapy); elevated troponin is associated with RV overdistension, pulmonary embolism, or ischemia.
2. EKG can detect right ventricular enlargement, right bundle branch block, right ventricular strain pattern, and S1Q3T3 pattern.
3. Chest X-ray can detect right ventricular enlargement and engorged pulmonary arteries.
4. Doppler echocardiography will help assess severity of pulmonary arterial hypertension.

TREATMENT

1. Identify and treat precipitating factors: SVT, sepsis, and pulmonary embolism.
2. SVT is triggered by hypervolemia or right heart dilation; avoid β-blockers and calcium channel inhibitors if possible, as they have a negative right ventricular inotropic effect; instead, consider converting pharmacologically with amiodaron[2] under anticoagulation.
3. Assess patients for infection:
   - Patients on IV prostacyclin have high risk for catheter-associated bacteremia; therefore, insidious sepsis due to *Micrococcus* or *Staphylococcus epidermidis* can trigger right heart failure.[3]
   - Patients may have bacterial translocation from the gut due to the combination of decreased cardiac output and increased venous pressure.[4]
4. Urgent surgical/catheter thrombectomy or systemic thrombolysis in patients with acute pulmonary embolism with hemodynamic instability.
5. Doppler echocardiography will help to assess response to treatment.[5]
6. Monitor right ventricular function with right heart or pulmonary artery catheterization; this will provide direct measurement of pulmonary artery pressure, cardiac output, and pulmonary vascular resistance and also will allow assessment of response to vasodilator therapy.
7. Continuous IV epoprostenol has the highest level of recommendation with evidence of survival benefit[6]:
   - Epoprostenol 2 ng/kg/min IV infusion pump over 24–48 h; titrate by 1–2 ng/kg/min q 15 min, until desired effect or dose-limiting pharmacologic effects occur.[7]
8. Inhaled nitric oxide dilates pulmonary vasculature, improves ventilation/perfusion match, reduces pulmonary artery pressure, and improves cardiac output; discontinue gradually to prevent rebound pulmonary hypertension.[8]
9. Other recommended medications (lower strength of recommendation compared to epoprostenol):
   - Treprostinil (inhaled, IV, or subcutaneous) reduces pulmonary vascular resistance and pulmonary artery pressure and improves right ventricular performance.
   - Iloprost (inhaled or IV) reduces pulmonary vascular resistance and pulmonary artery pressure and improves right ventricular performance.
   - Sildenafil (inhaled or IV) decreases pulmonary vascular resistance and pulmonary artery hypertension and improves cardiac output.[9]
10. Utilize vasopressors for hemodynamic support to maintain MAP of 60–65 mmHg:
    - Use norepinephrine 0.2 μg/kg/min; titrate up to 3.3 μg/kg/min.[10]
11. Utilize inotropes to decrease afterload and increase cardiac output:
    - Dobutamine in a range of 2–20 μg/kg/min[11]
    - Milrinone in a range of 0.3–0.75 μg/kg/min[12]
12. Intubation with mechanical ventilation, volume controlled, low tidal volume, plateau pressure < 27–30 mmHg.[9]
13. Refractory cases will require extracorporeal life support as a bridge to urgent heart or heart-lung transplantation.

References

1. Dunlap B, Weyer G. Pulmonary hypertension: diagnosis and treatment. *Am Fam Physician.* 2016; 94(6):463–469.
2. Vardas PE, Kochiadakis GE, Igoumenidis NE, et al. Amiodarone as a first choice drug for restoring sinus rhythm in patients with atrial fibrillation: a randomized, controlled study. *Chest.* 2000;117:1538–1545.

3. Boucly A, O'Connell C, Savale L, et al. Tunneled central venous line-associated infections in patients with pulmonary arterial hypertension treated with intravenous prostacyclin. *Presse Med.* 2016;45:20–28.
4. Hoeper MM, Granton J. Intensive care unit management of patients with severe pulmonary hypertension and right heart failure. *Am J Respir Crit Care Med.* 2011;184:1114–1124.
5. Hui-li G. The management of acute pulmonary arterial hypertension. *Cardiovasc Ther.* 2011;29:153–175.
6. Galiè N, Corris PA, Frost AE, et al. Updated treatment algorithm of pulmonary arterial hypertension. *J Am Coll Cardiol.* 2013;62(25):D60–D72.
7. *Epoprostenol.* Reference.medscape.com.
8. George I, Xydas S, Topkara VK, et al. Clinical indication for use and outcomes after inhaled nitric oxide therapy. *Ann Thorac Surg.* 2006;82:2161–2169.
9. Corris P, Degano B. Severe pulmonary arterial hypertension: treatment options and the bridge to transplantation. *Eur Respir Rev.* 2014;23:488–497.
10. *Norepinephrine.* Reference.medscape.com.
11. *Dobutamine.* Reference.medscape.com.
12. *Milrinone.* Reference.medscape.com.

Anaphylaxis

Presentation

Severe life-threatening systemic allergic reaction, for example, to food or medication. Medication-related anaphylaxis is more common in adults 55 or older. Radiocontrast media can also cause anaphylaxis. It usually occurs as a result of IgE-mediated response within 1 h of exposure to inciting agent.[1]

Anaphylaxis is most commonly manifested with acute respiratory and cardiovascular failure and dermatologic, gastrointestinal, and even neurological symptoms. Patients may develop throat constriction, tongue and lips edema, difficulty speaking, dysphagia, cough, voice changes, stridor, chest tightness, nausea, vomiting, abdominal cramps, and urticarial rash/hives.[1]

Causes for Rapid Response Activation

Worsening dyspnea, wheezing, tachypnea, stridor, cyanosis, tongue and lips edema, tachycardia, hypotension, altered mental status.

Actions

INITIAL MEASURES

1. STOP administering inciting drug.
2. Continuous pulse oximetry.
3. Administer 100% oxygen via nonrebreather mask or a one-way valve facemask with oxygen inlet port, usually 8–10 L/min.
4. Maintain continuous cardiac monitoring.
5. Have the patient lie in a recumbent position with lower extremities raised.
6. Ventilate with a bag/valve/mask until standard rapid sequence intubation (RSI) can be done in patients with airway compromise.
7. Consult anesthesiologist early for fiberoptic intubation; if not effective, cricothyrotomy or catheter jet ventilation must be done.

TREATMENT

1. Inject intramuscular (more rapid and reliable absorption than subcutaneous) epinephrine (1:1000 dilution) at 0.5 mg in the anterolateral thigh (vastus lateralis) every 5–15 min × 3 until adequate response is achieved (upper airway obstruction and hypotension resolved); onset of action is 3–5 min; epinephrine causes vasoconstriction, increased peripheral resistance, increased cardiac inotropy and chronotropy, bronchodilation, and decreased mucosal edema.[2]
2. If no adequate response to IM epinephrine occurs, start vasopressors such as epinephrine (1:10,000 dilution) at 1–10 μg/min.[2]
3. Use IV normal saline or lactated ringer at 1 L boluses through two large-bore catheters for hypotensive patients; usually 2 L is administered initially; large volumes of crystalloid may

be required, potentially exceeding 5 L; if hypotension is refractory, place central venous catheter and arterial line.[2]

4. Maintain continuous albuterol nebulizer for patients with bronchospasm:
   - Albuterol 2.5 mg nebulized every 4 h as needed[3]
5. Administer racemic epinephrine nebulizer for patients with laryngeal edema:
   - Racemic epinephrine 0.5 mL of 2.25% solution diluted in 3 mL NS via jet nebulizer every 4 h as needed[4]
6. For hypotensive patients taking beta-blockers, administer glucagon 3.5–5 mg IV; repeat in 10 min if no improved blood pressure response.[2]
7. Administer diphenhydramine 25–50 mg IV to improve cutaneous erythema and decrease pruritus; it does not reverse airway obstruction or hypotension; onset of action is 1–2 h.[2]
8. Famotidine 20 mg IV causes improved response compared to diphenhydramine used alone.
9. Administer hydrocortisone 250 mg IV to prevent recurrent reaction; onset of action is 6 h after administration.[2]

References

1. Arnold JJ, Williams PM. Anaphylaxis: recognition and management. *Am Fam Physician.* 2011; 84(10):1111–1118.
2. Tang AW. A practical guide to anaphylaxis. *Am Fam Physician.* 2003;68(7):1325–1333.
3. *Albuterol.* Reference.medscape.com.
4. *Racemic Epinephrine.* Reference.medscape.com.

Acute Nonhistaminergic Angioedema

Presentation

Acute respiratory failure due to nonhistaminergic angioedema is characterized by bradykinin-mediated angioedema. Etiologies include ACE inhibitors (e.g., lisinopril), hereditary angioedema (C1-INH deficiency), acquired angioedema (C1-INH deficiency, e.g., in lymphoma or monoclonal gammopathy), and estrogen-dependent angioedema due to decreased functional C1-INH.

Angioedema is nonpruritic and nonpitting edema and can involve any part of the body, including face, frequently lips and tongue, pharynx, larynx, hands, feet, abdomen, gluteal area, and genitalia.[1] Patients may experience pain and dysesthesias such as numbness, tingling, and burning in the affected areas, dysphonia, dysphagia, nausea, vomiting, diarrhea, and abdominal pain. These patients will not have urticaria.

Causes for Rapid Response Activation

Laryngeal edema with symptoms of hoarseness, stridor, asphyxia.

Actions

1. STOP administering inciting drug (e.g., lisinopril).
2. Continuous pulse oximetry/capnography.
3. 100% oxygen via nonrebreather mask, usually 8–10 L/min.
4. Nasal trumpets may act as temporizing measures and may assist with bag-valve mask ventilation.
5. Ventilate with a bag/valve/mask until standard rapid sequence intubation (RSI) can be done in patients with airway compromise.
6. Maintain continuous cardiac monitoring.
7. Have the patient lie in a recumbent position with lower extremities raised.

DIAGNOSTIC WORK-UP

1. Labs: C4; if low, proceed with C1-INH level, C1-INH function, and C1q level.
2. In stable patients with abdominal symptoms, perform CT scan of abdomen and pelvis to check for presence of dilated bowel loops, thickened mucosal folds, bowel edema, perihepatic edema, and ascites.

TREATMENT

1. Airway protection is the most important component of management; therefore, consult a pulmonologist, an otolaryngologist, or an anesthesiologist early in the course of treatment, as intubation with mechanical ventilation may be indicated.

2. Fiberoptic intubation may be indicated in patients with a difficult airway.
3. In severe laryngeal edema or when fiberoptic intubation is not effective, consult surgeon for cricothyrotomy or tracheotomy.[2]
4. Antihistamines or corticosteroids do not work in nonhistaminergic angioedema.[2]
5. For adult patients with hereditary angioedema, including pregnant and breast-feeding patients, administer plasma-derived C1-INH 20U/kg IV; 68% of patients will have improvement of symptoms within 1h after administration and 87% within 4h after administration.[2]
6. For patients with hereditary angioedema (no pregnancy safety data is available), you can also use one of the two FDA-approved C-1 esterase inhibitor concentrates as soon as angioedema is recognized:
   - Ecallantide (kallikrein inhibitor) 30mg (3mL) SC administered in three separate 10mg (1mL) injections; if attack persists, you may administer an additional dose of 30mg within 24h.
   - Icatibant (bradykinin B2 receptor antagonist) 30mg SC × 3 in abdominal area, not to exceed a total of three injections within 24h.[3]
7. Fresh frozen plasma (FFP) contains C1-INH; administer 2 units, if other therapies are not available; as FFP may potentially contain substrates that can worsen angioedema, administer FFP in ICU setting and be ready to intubate and mechanically ventilate the patient.[2]
8. Tranexamic acid 1g IV can be administered if other therapies are not available.
9. Consult allergy specialist when patient is stable.

References

1. Muller BA. Urticaria and angioedema: a practical approach. *Am Fam Physician.* 2004;69(5):1123–1129.
2. Li HH, Kaliner MA. *Angioedema Treatment and Management.* Emedicine.medscape.com. Updated: September 04, 2018.
3. Powell RJ, Leech SC, Till S, et al. BSACI guideline for the management of chronic urticaria and angioedema. *Clin Exp Allergy.* 2015;45(3):547–565.

CHAPTER 3

Neurological Emergencies

Seizure/Status Epilepticus

Presentation

Status epilepticus is a common life-threatening neurological emergency. The Epilepsy Foundation working group recommended that emergency department physicians define seizures as status epilepticus if seizure activity continues for more than 10 min.[1]

Presentations include new onset seizure disorder or exacerbation of preexisting seizure disorder. It is easily recognized in patients with general convulsions; however, patients with nonconvulsive presentation require higher index of suspicion.

Change of medication is the most common trigger in patients with known seizure disorder. Other precipitating factors include infection, brain tumors, metabolic disorders, alcohol withdrawal, sleep deprivation, illicit drugs, or toxic ingestions.[2]

Causes for Rapid Response Activation

Any type of seizure, including generalized tonic-clonic seizures and subtle seizures, impaired consciousness, hypotension, aspiration, respiratory failure.

Actions

INITIAL MEASURES

1. Continuous pulse oximetry.
2. Supplemental oxygen to maintain $SpO_2 > 92\%$ or $PaO_2 > 60$–$65\,mmHg$; transition to high flow oxygen when patient requires high flow rates.
3. Continuous cardiac monitoring.
4. Seizure/fall precautions.
5. Establish large-bore IV access if patient does not already have one.

DIAGNOSTIC WORK-UP

1. ABG allows assessment of hypoxia and metabolic acidosis.
2. Labs: CBC with differential (elevated WBC in infection), procalcitonin (elevated in bacterial or fungal infection), BMP, magnesium, liver panel, toxicologic screening, serum pregnancy test in women of childbearing age, and antiepileptic medications levels.
3. UA, urine, blood and sputum cultures in patients with suspected infection.
4. Order EKG to identify cardiac arrhythmias that could potentially lead to cerebral hypoperfusion or atrial fibrillation that could potentially cause a thromboembolic stroke.

5. Order electroencephalography (EEG); for patients with new-onset seizure, the sooner the EEG is done after seizure, the higher the chance of seizure detection; tonic, clonic, or tonic-clonic seizures can be dramatic initially and then may evolve into subtle movements such as twitching of the limb, face, or eyelid, which should not be misinterpreted as improvement, and treatment should continue until resolution of seizure electrical activity on EEG.[3]

6. If available, continuous EEG for paralyzed patients, intubated patients, and patients with refractory status epilepticus.[3]

7. After patient is stabilized, order noncontrast head CT scan to evaluate for structural lesions such as a brain tumor, an infarct, a hemorrhage, or an abscess.

8. Lumbar puncture is reserved for patients with persistent fever, altered mental status, headache, and for immunocompromised patients.

TREATMENT

1. Check glucose level (both hyperglycemia and hypoglycemia can be associated with status epilepticus); if hypoglycemic, administer 50 mL bolus of 50% dextrose IV.[2]

2. Consider thiamine 100 mg IV.

3. The following three phases of treatment are outlined in the American Epilepsy Society's 2016 guidelines for the treatment of status epilepticus[4,5]:

   First-line agents:
   - o Lorazepam 2 mg IV per minute, normally 0.1 mg/kg in total; however, there is no specific upper limit for benzodiazepines; sometimes large doses may be needed.
   - o Diazepam 5–10 mg IV per minute.
   - o Midazolam 5 mg spray into one nostril; if patients do not respond after 10 min, administer additional 5 mg spray into the opposite nostril.

   Second-line agents for patients who continue to seize ≥ 5 min despite aggressive benzodiazepine treatment:
   - ▪ Fosphenytoin 15–20 mg PE/kg IV at a rate of 100–150 mg PE/min; monitor for arrhythmias and hypotension; check the level 2 h after the loading dose, with the goal being a level of 15–20 μg/mL.
   - ▪ Valproic acid 20 mg/kg IV over 10 min; the goal blood level is 100 μg/mL, and blood can be drawn immediately after the loading dose has been administered; contraindicated in hepatic dysfunction.
   - ▪ Levetiracetam 1-3 g IV over 15 min; adjust the dose to renal function.
   - ▪ Phenobarbital 20 mg/kg IV at a rate of 50–100 mg/min; monitor respiration status and blood pressure.

   Third-line agents for patients who still continue to seize ≥ 20 min should be given after these patients are intubated:
   - ▪ Propofol infusion 2–5 mg/kg bolus, followed by 20–200 μg/kg/min infusion.
   - ▪ Midazolam infusion 0.01–0.05 mg/kg bolus, followed by 0.02–0.1 mg/kg/h infusion.
   - ▪ Pentobarbital 5–15 mg/kg bolus, followed by 0.5–1 mg/kg/h infusion.

References

1. Treatment of convulsive status epilepticus. Recommendations of the Epilepsy Foundation of America's Working Group on Status Epilepticus. *JAMA*. 1993;270(7):854–859.
2. Roth JL. *Status Epilepticus Treatment and Management*. Emedicine.medscape.com. Updated: December 23, 2020.
3. Yigit O, Eray O, Mihci E, Yilmaz D, Eray B, Ozkaynak S. EEG as a part of decision-making process in the emergency department. *Eur J Emerg Med*. 2013;20(6):402–407.
4. Glauser T, Shinnar S, Gloss D, et al. Treatment of convulsive status epilepticus in children and adults: report of the guideline committee of the American Epilepsy Society. *Epilepsy Curr*. 2016;16(1):48–61.
5. Falco-Walter JJ, Bleck T. Treatment of established status epilepticus. *J Clin Med*. 2016;5(5):49.

Acute Ischemic Stroke

Presentation

Acute ischemic stroke is a sudden onset of neurological deficit that occurs due to sudden loss of blood circulation to an area of the brain. It is caused by thrombotic or embolic blockage of the cerebral artery.

Symptoms include but are not limited to motor deficits (hemiparesis, monoparesis, quadriparesis), sensory deficits, monocular or binocular vision loss, visual field deficits, diplopia, dysarthria, facial droop, ataxia, aphasia, and sudden decrease in the level of consciousness.

Causes for Code Stroke Activation

Symptoms and signs of stroke.

Actions

INITIAL MEASURES

1. Continuous pulse oximetry.
2. Supplemental oxygen for hypoxic patients to maintain $SpO_2 > 94\%$.
3. Continuous cardiac and blood pressure monitoring.
4. Perform brief and accurate neurological examination to identify neurological deficits and to localize the lesion.
5. Assess the severity of stroke according to NIHSS (National Institutes of Health Stroke Scale); initial NIHSS predicts functional outcome.
6. Establish the time of symptom onset or the time at which the patient was last known normal.

DIAGNOSTIC WORK-UP

1. The only required tests for eligibility of the patient for IV alteplase are:
   - Serum glucose level, as hypoglycemia may be a stroke mimic
   - Noncontrast head CT within 20 min of arrival (onset of symptoms) to exclude intracranial hemorrhage before IV alteplase administration
   - If coagulopathy is suspected, INR, PTT, and platelet count
2. Consider other labs: CBC (polycythemia, thrombocytosis), BMP (hypoglycemia, hyponatremia), troponin, and serum pregnancy test for all women of childbearing age.
3. Order EKG.
4. Telemetry for at least 24 h to screen for arrhythmias such as atrial fibrillation.

TREATMENT

1. Correct hypotension and hypovolemia to maintain adequate systemic perfusion of organs.
2. In hypertensive patients eligible for treatment with IV alteplase and/or mechanical thrombectomy, blood pressures should be carefully lowered to < 185/110 mmHg before treatment, using one of the following agents:

- Nicardipine 5 mg/h IV, titrating up by 2.5 mg/h every 5–15 min, with maximum dose 15 mg/h
- Clevidipine 1–2 mg/h IV, titrating up by doubling the dose every 2–5 min, with maximum dose 21 mg/h
- Labetalol 10–20 mg over 1–2 min; may repeat one time

3. Door-to-needle time for IV alteplase should ideally be < 60 min.
4. IV alteplase should be administered to the following patients:
   - Patients with ischemic stroke causing measurable neurological deficit
   - Eligible patients within 3 h after the onset of stroke symptoms or last known normal
   - Selective group of eligible patients based on European Cooperative Acute Stroke Study (ECASS) III exclusion criteria within 4.5 h after the onset of stroke symptoms or last known normal
5. Exclusion criteria for IV alteplase within 3 h after the onset of stroke symptoms:
   - Mild nondisabling stroke symptoms
   - Rapidly improving stroke symptoms and disability
   - Blood pressure ≥ 185/110
   - Hypoglycemia with blood glucose < 50
   - Acute intracranial hemorrhage on CT scan of head
   - Previous history of intracranial hemorrhage
   - Current subarachnoid hemorrhage
   - Recent (within 3 months) ischemic stroke
   - Recent (within 3 months) severe head trauma
   - Recent (within 3 months) intracranial or intraspinal surgery
   - GI malignancy or GI bleeding within 21 days
   - Coagulopathy: platelets < 100,000 mm^3, INR > 1.7, aPTT > 40 s, or PT > 15 s
   - Full treatment dose of LMWH within previous 24 h
   - Direct oral anticoagulants within last 48 h
   - Suspected or confirmed endocarditis
   - Intra-axial intracranial neoplasm
   - Aortic arch dissection
6. ECASS-III exclusion criteria for IV alteplase within 4.5 h after the onset of stroke symptoms:
   - Age > 80 years
   - Severe stroke with NIHSS > 25
   - History of diabetes mellitus and prior stroke
   - Taking an oral anticoagulant regardless of INR
   - Imaging evidence of ischemic injury involving > 1/3 of the MCA territory
7. Administer alteplase infusion 0.9 mg/kg (maximum dose 90 mg), over 60 min, with 10% of the dose given as a bolus over 1 min in ICU.
8. Check blood pressure and perform neurological assessment q 15 min during and after IV alteplase infusion for 2 h, then every 30 min for 6 h, then hourly until 24 h after IV alteplase treatment.
9. Discontinue IV alteplase and obtain emergency noncontrast CT scan of head if patient has the following issues:
   - Severe headache, nausea, or vomiting
   - Acute hypertension
   - Worsening neurological status
10. Obtain follow-up CT scan or MRI of head at 24 h after IV alteplase before starting antiplatelet agent or anticoagulant.

11. Order urgent CTA with CTP or MRA with DW MRI with or without MR perfusion to assess for large vessel occlusion.

12. Mechanical thrombectomy with a stent retriever is indicated for the following cases:
    - Causative occlusion of ICA or proximal MCA
    - NIHSS ≥ 6
    - Reassuring noncontrast head CT with ASPECT (Alberta Stroke Program Early Computed Tomography) score ≥ 6
    - Within 6 h of last known normal
    - Patients ≥ 18 years

13. Start aspirin within 24–48 h after stroke onset, unless patients are eligible for IV alteplase, in which case delay aspirin for 24 h.

14. In patients with minor (NIHSS ≤ 3) noncardioembolic ischemic stroke who did not receive IV alteplase, start dual antiplatelet therapy (aspirin and clopidogrel) within 24 h after symptom onset and continue for 21 days; this treatment is effective in reducing recurrent ischemic stroke for a period of up to 90 days from symptom onset.

15. Treat hypoglycemic patients (blood sugar < 60 mg/dL) with 50 mL bolus of 50% dextrose IV.

16. Treat hyperglycemia to achieve blood glucose levels in a range of 140–180 mg/dL.

17. In patients with large cerebral or cerebellar stroke with high risk for brain swelling and herniation (decreasing level of consciousness, neurological deterioration within 48 h despite medical therapy), consult neurosurgery for the following measures:
    - Decompressive craniectomy with dural expansion, which is reasonable in patients ≤ 60 and can be considered in patients > 60
    - Osmotic therapy
    - Brief moderate hyperventilation with pCO_2 target of 30–34 mmHg

18. Secondary stroke prevention:
    - The effectiveness of routine echocardiogram for secondary stroke prevention in all patients with acute ischemic stroke is uncertain.
    - Screen all patients with acute ischemic stroke for diabetes mellitus with HgA1C.
    - Initiate oral anticoagulation for embolic stroke in the setting of atrial fibrillation between 4–14 days after the onset of stroke symptoms.
    - Screen for and treat hyperlipidemia.
    - Optimize treatment of hypertension.
    - Smoking cessation.

Further Reading

1. Power WJ, Rabinstein AA, Ackerson T, et al. Guidelines for the early management of patients with acute ischemic stroke: 2019 update to 2018 guidelines for the early management of acute ischemic stroke: a guideline for healthcare professionals from the American Heart Association/American Stroke Association. *Stroke.* 2019;50:e344–e418.

Acute Hemorrhagic Stroke

Presentation

Patients with vascular comorbidities such as prior ischemic or hemorrhagic stroke, hypertension, diabetes mellitus, and who smoke are at high risk. Symptoms and signs include sudden focal neurological deficit that progresses over minutes to hours, headache, vomiting, decreased level of consciousness, elevated systolic blood pressure > 220 mmHg, and coma. Carotid endarterectomy or carotid stenting increase hyperperfusion and subsequent risk for hemorrhagic stroke.

Causes for Rapid Response Activation

Symptoms and signs of stroke.

Actions

INITIAL MEASURES

1. Continuous pulse oximetry.
2. Supplemental oxygen to maintain $SpO_2 > 94\%$.
3. Continuous cardiac and blood pressure monitoring with cycled automated BP cuff.
4. Establish the time of symptom onset or the time at which the patient was last known normal.
5. Perform brief and accurate neurological examination to identify neurological deficits and to localize the lesion.
6. Assess the severity of stroke according to ICH (Intracerebral Hemorrhage) score or NIHSS (National Institutes of Health Stroke Scale). Initial ICH score and NIHSS predict functional outcome.

DIAGNOSTIC WORK-UP

1. Labs: CBC, BMP, coagulation studies (PT, INR, aPTT), troponin, toxicology screen to detect cocaine or other stimulants, urinalysis, and urine pregnancy test in women of childbearing age.
2. Order EKG to assess for ischemia or arrhythmias.
3. Order head CT scan or MRI to distinguish ischemic stroke from intracranial hemorrhage.
4. Consider CTA and contrast-enhanced CT to identify patients at risk for hematoma expansion, such as presence of contrast within hematoma, termed the contrast spot sign.
5. Consider CTA and contrast-enhanced CT; CT venography; contrast-enhanced MRI, MRA, and MR venography; and catheter angiography to better identify causes of hemorrhage, such as AVM, tumors, moyamoya, or cerebral vein thrombosis.

TREATMENT

1. Discontinue all anticoagulants and antiplatelet agents.
2. Administer reversal anticoagulants and antiplatelet agents:
   - IV heparin infusion or subcutaneous heparin-protamine 1 mg/100 U of heparin; maximum dose is 50 mg IV.

- Subcutaneous enoxaparin (Lovenox)-protamine 0.5–1 mg/1 mg of enoxaparin; maximum dose is 50 mg IV.
- Fondaparinux (Arixtra) (factor Xa inhibitor)-rFVIIa (NovoSeven) 90 µg/kg IV.
- Warfarin-vitamin K 10 mg IV given slowly over 30 min (onset of action in 2 h and is maximal at 24 h) and FFP 2–4 units or prothrombin complex concentrate (PCC), activated PCC FEIBA (factor VIII inhibitor bypassing activity), or recombinant activated factor VIIa; target INR < 1.3–1.5.
- Dabigatran (Pradaxa) (direct thrombin inhibitor)-idarucizumab (Praxbind); infuse 5 g dose IV as two consecutive 2.5 g infusions, a monoclonal antibody that directly targets dabigatran—treatment approved by FDA in 2015; if idarucizumab is not available, consider 4-factor PCC (KCentra) 25–50 IU/kg; consider hemodialysis in patients with renal impairment.
- Rivaroxaban (Xarelto) or apixaban (Eliquis) (factor Xa inhibitors)-andexanet (Andexxa) 400–800 mg IV depending on the dose and timing of the last dose—treatment approved by FDA in 2018; if andexanet is not available, consider 4-factor PCC (KCentra) 25–50 IU/kg.
- Activated charcoal 50–100 g via nasogastric tube may be administered if the ingestion is within 2–6 h for dabigatran, apixaban, and rivaroxaban.

3. In hypertensive patients, reduce blood pressure acutely to the goal of 140 mmHg with:
   - Nicardipine drip 5 mg/h by slow infusion initially; may be increased by 2.5 mg/h every 15 min, not to exceed 15 mg/h.
4. Monitor glucose to avoid both hyperglycemia and hypoglycemia.
5. Fever is common in patients with intracerebral hemorrhage, especially in patients with intraventricular hemorrhage, and they should be treated with antipyretics such as rectal acetaminophen.
6. Patients with intracerebral hemorrhage are at high risk for seizures, especially patients with cortical involvement of the hemorrhage; the majority of seizures occur at or near the onset of the hemorrhage; seizures should be treated with antiseizure medications.
7. An EEG is recommended for patients with depressed mental status; if the EEG shows electrographic evidence of seizure, these patients should be treated with antiseizure medications.
8. Administer thromboprophylaxis (intermittent pneumatic compression together with elastic stockings); after cessation of bleeding, discuss with neurosurgeon whether you can start low dose of subcutaneous low-molecular-weight heparin or unfractionated heparin in patients with lack of mobility.
9. If Glasgow Coma Scale (GCS) is 3–8, intubate; if GCS is > 8, do not intubate and allow neurosurgeon to make assessment.
10. Monitor intracranial pressure (ICP) in patients with GCS of 3–8 and clinical evidence of transtentorial herniation, significant intraventricular hemorrhage, or hydrocephalus; ICP is measured by ventricular catheter inserted into the brain parenchyma or cerebral ventricle; increased ICP is more common in younger patients and patients with supratentorial hemorrhage.
11. Ventricular catheter inserted into the lateral ventricle can also be used for therapeutic purposes to drain cerebrospinal fluid (CSF) and to reduce ICP; goal ICP is < 20 mmHg, and goal CPP (cerebral perfusion pressure) is 60–70 mmHg.
12. Treat elevated ICP (please see a chapter on Acute Intracranial Hypertension).
13. Decompressive craniectomy with hematoma evacuation is indicated for patients with cerebellar hemorrhage who are deteriorating neurologically or who have brainstem compression or hydrocephalus from ventricular obstruction.

14. Decompressive craniectomy with or without hematoma evacuation may reduce mortality in patients with supratentorial hemorrhage who are deteriorating neurologically, large hematomas with significant midline shift, or elevated ICP refractory to medical management.

15. All patients should have a formal screening protocol for dysphagia before initiation of oral intake.

Further Reading

Hemphill III JC, Greenberg SM, Anderson CS, et al. Guidelines for the management of spontaneous intracerebral hemorrhage. A guideline for healthcare professionals from the American Heart Association/American Stroke Association. *Stroke*. 2015;46:2032–2060.

Acute Intracranial Hypertension

Presentation

Acute increase in intracranial pressure (normal ICP is 5–15 mmHg)[1] can occur in patients with acute intraventricular, intraparenchymal, subarachnoid, epidural or subdural hematomas, severe hydrocephalus, severe brain traumas, brain tumors, and severe ischemic strokes.

Patients with acute intracranial hypertension (defined as ICP > 20 mmHg)[1] may have headache, nausea, vomiting, somnolence, blurry vision, double vision, focal neurologic deficits progressing to herniation syndrome (e.g., pupillary changes, cranial nerve, especially the third and sixth, nerve palsies), and worsening paresis. Patients may have Cushing's triad: bradycardia, irregular respirations, and widened pulse pressure. Patients with acute increase in ICP will usually have low GCS score. In comatose patients, papilledema is a reliable sign of intracranial hypertension.[2]

Causes for Rapid Response Activation

Worsening altered mental status, severe bradycardia, acute hypoxic/hypercapnic respiratory distress, motor posturing, hypotension.

Actions

INITIAL MEASURES

1. Continuous pulse oximetry.
2. Supplemental oxygen to maintain $SpO_2 \geq 94\%$.
3. Continuous cardiac and blood pressure monitoring.
4. Elevate head of bed to 15–30 degrees, which is associated with significant decrease in ICP and assure neutral and midline position of the head to keep jugular veins open.
5. Consult with neurosurgeon early in the course of the rapid response.

TREATMENT

1. Control pain with opioid analgesics (e.g., IV morphine) and agitation with benzodiazepines (e.g., IV lorazepam), as pain and agitation can increase intracranial pressure.
2. Control fever with antipyretics such as rectal acetaminophen and cooling blankets.
3. Control hypertension with medications that reduce systemic hypertension without affecting ICP and with short half-life, for example:
   - Esmolol loading dose 500 µg/kg IV over 1 min, followed by 50 µg/kg/min; titrate to maximum of 200 µg/kg/min.[3]
   - Labetalol 20 mg IV bolus; may repeat doses of 20–80 mg IV at 10 min intervals until goal blood pressure is achieved, with maximum 24 h total of 300 mg[3]; dose reduction may be needed in hepatic impairment.
4. In patients with primary or metastatic brain tumors, may use steroids, such as dexamethasone 4 mg IV every 6 h; otherwise, avoid steroids, especially in cases of traumatic brain injury.

5. Treat seizures with antiepileptics.

6. Consult neurosurgery for ventricular catheter placement through a burr hole to monitor ICP, which can also be used for therapeutic CSF drainage; the catheter should be checked for proper functioning every 2–4 h and any time there is a change in the ICP, CSF output, or neuro examination.[4]

7. Hyperventilation causes a decrease in pCO_2 with subsequent cerebral arteriolar constriction and reduced cerebral blood volume, which leads to a decrease in ICP; the effect lasts for < 24 h, and prolonged hyperventilation should be avoided.[1]

8. Administer mannitol as an initial bolus of 0.25–1 g/kg IV; this can be repeated at 0.25–0.5 g/kg IV doses every 6–8 h as needed; renal toxicity is one of the primary concerns; therefore, check serum osmolarity to calculate osmolar gap (osmolar gap = measured serum osmolarity − calculated serum osmolarity), goal osmolar gap is < 18–20; other concerns include extravasation and fluid-electrolyte imbalance.[5]

9. Order IV fluids such as crystalloids to maintain euvolemia, as mannitol may cause urinary osmotic diuresis and decrease plasma osmolarity.

10. If patient is refractory to mannitol, a 3%–23.4% hypertonic saline can be used as 30–60 mL IV bolus over 15 min.[6]

11. In patients with intractable shivering, posturing, or agitation, neuromuscular blockade with nondepolarizing agent; for example, vecuronium and intubation can be used.

12. Consult with neurosurgery regarding surgical interventions, for example, drainage of brain abscess, evacuation of pneumocephalus, drainage of CSF, resection of intracranial tumor, decompressive craniectomy for neurologically deteriorating patients refractory to mannitol.

13. In patients who are refractory to medical and surgical management, pentobarbital may be considered as a bolus of 10–30 mg/kg followed by 0.5–3 mg/kg/h, titrated to a serum level of 30–50 µg/mL or until the electroencephalogram shows a burst suppression pattern; may need concomitant use of IV fluid and vasopressor, as barbiturates cause cardiac suppression and vasodilatation.[1]

References

1. Zakaria A, Aisiku IP. Management of acute intracranial hypertension. *Critical Care. Emergency Medicine.* 2nd ed. McGrawHill Education; vol. 32; 2017:335–339.
2. Kamel H, Hemphill III JC. Characteristics and sequelae of intracranial hypertension after intracerebral hemorrhage. *Neurocrit Care.* 2012;17:172–176.
3. Levy ZD, Zhou Q, Slesinger TL. Hypertensive crises. *Critical Care. Emergency Medicine.* 2nd ed. McGrawHill Education; vol. 17; 2017:175–183.
4. Rangel-Castillo L, Gopinath S, Robertson CS. Management of intracranial hypertension. *Neurol Clin.* 2008;26(2):521–541.
5. *Mannitol (Systemic).* Drugs.com.
6. Rockswold GL, et al. Hypertonic saline and its effect on intracranial pressure, cerebral perfusion pressure, and brain tissue oxygen. *Neurosurgery.* 2009;65(6):1035–1104.

Delirium/Agitation in Intensive Care Unit/Hospital Wards

Presentation

Delirium is an impaired cognition with a variety of neuropsychiatric symptoms and signs and may be associated with long-term cognitive dysfunction. Delirium most frequently occurs in hospitalized elderly patients, patients with dementia, mechanically ventilated patients, and patients with alcohol abuse. Other risk factors include living alone; smoking > 10 cigarettes/day; acute illness such as severe sepsis; medications such as antihistamines, anticholinergics, corticosteroids, metoclopramide, opiates, and benzodiazepines; and malnutrition.[1]

Delirium is classified as hyperactive (agitated and restless), hypoactive (lethargic and apathetic), or mixed type. Hypoactive delirium is more frequent in patients admitted to ICU, is often missed, and is associated with greater need for mechanical ventilation, prolonged ICU stay, and increased mortality, compared to hyperactive delirium.[1]

Symptoms may include disorientation, reduced attentiveness, reduced awareness of the environment, memory impairment, dysarthria, hallucinations, and delusions.[2] Symptoms tend to fluctuate.

Causes for Rapid Response Activation

Severely agitated patient with hallucinations, delusions, or combative behavior with potential injury to self or others.

Actions

INITIAL MEASURES

1. Assess patient's level of consciousness with Richmond Agitation Sedation Scale (RASS).[1]
2. Screen the patient for delirium using one of the following:
   - Confusion Assessment Method for the Intensive Care Unit (CAM–ICU)
   - Intensive Care Delirium Screening Checklist (ICDSC)[1]
3. Discontinue drugs associated with delirium.

DIAGNOSTIC WORK-UP

1. Labs: CBC with differential (leukocytosis in infection, low hemoglobin in anemia), procalcitonin (elevated in bacterial and fungal infection), BMP (electrolyte abnormalities, impaired renal function, hypoglycemia), liver function tests, thyroid function tests, urinalysis (UTI), thiamine level, B12 level, and urine drug screen.
2. Order chest X-ray to assess for pneumonia, pleural effusion, or pulmonary vascular congestion.
3. Order CT scan of head or MRI of head in patients with suspected ischemic or hemorrhagic stroke or structural lesions.

4. Order EEG in patients with suspected subtle seizures or nonconvulsive state.
5. Order lumbar puncture in patients with suspected CNS infection.

TREATMENT

1. Antipsychotics are the drugs of choice and should be used at the lowest adequate dosages, especially in elderly patients, and should be tapered down and discontinued once the delirium-precipitating condition is addressed and symptoms of delirium are under control[3]:
    - Administer haloperidol lactate 2–10 mg IV depending on the degree of agitation; if response is not satisfactory, repeat bolus q 15–30 min, sequentially doubling initial bolus dose; when patient becomes calm, administer 25% of last bolus dose every 6 h; taper dose after patient is controlled.[4]
    - If agitated patient loses IV access, administer haloperidol lactate 2–5 mg IM every 4–8 h PRN; may be required every hour in acute agitation; do not exceed 20 mg/day.[4]
    - Monitor EKG, as QT prolongation may occur with cumulative doses ≥ 35 mg and torsades de pointes with a single dose ≥ 20 mg, subsequently causing ventricular arrhythmias.[4]
    - Monitor other side effects such as dysphoria (dissatisfaction with life), extrapyramidal effects such as akathisia (restlessness, e.g., patient may fidget or rock back and forth), tardive dyskinesia, neuroleptic malignant syndrome, and dystonia (laryngospasm, trismus).[3]
2. Atypical antipsychotics have fewer extrapyramidal side effects:
    - Quetiapine (Seroquel) 25 mg orally twice daily
    - Olanzapine (Zyprexa) 2.5–5 mg orally daily
    - Risperidone (Risperdal) 0.25–0.5 mg orally twice daily[5]
3. Benzodiazepines are used in alcohol withdrawal delirium.
4. For patients with alcohol toxicity or withdrawal, administer thiamin 500 mg IV three times a day for two consecutive days, followed by 500 mg IV daily for 5 more days.[6]
5. Order continuous observation by one-to-one sitters.
6. Use soft mechanical restraints to prevent self-harm, such as self-extubation; removal of indwelling Foley catheters; removal of central venous catheters, arterial catheters, peripheral IV lines, and drains; and climbing out of bed and falling.
7. Identify and treat precipitating causes of delirium, such as infection, hypoxia, hypoglycemia, urinary retention, constipation, or fecal impaction.
8. Nonpharmacological therapies will help prevent delirium:
    - Correct dehydration.
    - Prevent sleep deprivation: use low-level lighting in the room, reduce the noise during sleep (ear plugs), discontinue the use of unnecessary monitors, adjust alarm volumes to the safest minimum level, avoid interventions during sleep hours, avoid caffeine at bedtime, and use scheduled melatonin.
    - For systematic orientation, place a clock and calendar in the room and reorient the patient frequently.
    - Provide eyeglasses and hearing aids.
    - Start early mobilization and early physical and occupational therapy.
    - Use therapeutic activities designed to lessen cognitive impairment.
    - Utilize the "wake up and breathe" protocol in critically ill patients requiring mechanical ventilation; the protocol uses a combination of the spontaneous awakening trial (SAT), such as interruption of sedation, and the spontaneous breathing trial (SBT).
    - Music therapy reduces anxiety.
    - Use sitters.
    - Engage family members and place family photos in the room.
    - Improve nutrition.[5]

References

1. Arumugam S, et al. Delirium in the intensive care unit. *J Emerg Trauma Shock.* 2017;10(1):37–46.
2. Markowitz JD, Narasimhan M. Delirium and antipsychotics: a systematic review of epidemiology and somatic treatment options. *Psychiatry.* 2008;5(10):29–36.
3. Alagiakrishnan K. *Delirium.* Emedicine.medscape.com. Updated: April 25, 2019.
4. *Haloperidol.* Reference.medscape.com.
5. Fosnight S, et al. *Delirium in the elderly. PSAP-VII. Geriatrics*; 2011:73–96.
6. Nishimoto A, et al. High dose parenteral thiamine in treatment of Wernicke's encephalopathy: case series and review of the literature. *In Vivo.* 2017;31(1):121–124.

Myasthenic Crisis

Presentation

Myasthenia gravis is an autoimmune neuromuscular disorder characterized by weakness of skeletal muscles. Muscle weakness occurs due to antibody-mediated attack directed at acetylcholine receptors on the postsynaptic membrane of the neuromuscular junction.

Myasthenic crisis can occur due to infection, noncompliance with medications, certain medications (e.g., antibiotics such as fluoroquinolones or macrolides, antipsychotics, β-blockers, calcium channel blockers, muscle relaxants, and contrast media), thyroid disorders, surgical procedures, emotional stressors. Patients develop specific painless muscle weakness that is worse with repeated use and better with rest.

Myasthenic crisis usually involves upper airway and respiratory muscles. Patients can have ptosis due to weakness of eyelid muscles, diplopia due to weakness of extraocular muscles, slurred or nasal speech due to facial muscle weakness, dysarthria, difficulty chewing and dysphagia due to the weakness of pharyngeal muscles, dyspnea, or difficulty sitting up or walking.[1]

Causes for Rapid Response Activation

Respiratory failure caused by aspiration of oral secretions due to bulbar muscle weakness or bronchospasm with dyspnea, wheezing, cyanosis due to respiratory muscle weakness.

Actions

INITIAL MEASURES

1. Continuous pulse oximetry.
2. Supplemental oxygen to maintain $SpO_2 > 92\%$ or $PaO_2 > 60\text{--}65\,mmHg$; transition to high flow oxygen when patient requires high flow rates.
3. Continuous cardiac monitoring.
4. Continuous capnography.
5. Check FVC (forced vital capacity) using spirometer at bedside (volume of exhaled air after maximal inspiration, normal is 60–70 mL/kg) while the patient is sitting up; FVC of 30 mL/kg is indicative of myasthenic crisis with airway compromise and necessitates transfer of the patient to ICU.[1]
6. Consult neurologist early in the course of crisis.

DIAGNOSTIC WORK-UP

1. Order ABG to assess severity of hypoxia or hypercapnia.
2. Labs: CBC (leukocytosis in infection), BMP (concomitant electrolyte abnormalities or impaired renal function), and magnesium.
3. Order chest X-ray to assess aspiration, lobar collapse, and pneumonia.

TREATMENT

1. Use cooling measures and antipyretics to lower temperature and improve muscle strength.
2. Position jaw and tongue, and suction pulmonary secretions.
3. Start BiPAP for patients with mild-to-moderate dyspnea who are able to clear secretions and protect their airway and are without overt hypercapnia; independent predictors of noninvasive ventilation (NIV) success are a serum bicarbonate $< 30\,mmol/L$ and an APACHE II score $< 6^2$; an independent predictor of noninvasive ventilation failure is hypercapnia with $PCO_2 > 45\,mmHg$.[3]
4. Ventilate by bag-valve mask while preparing to intubate.
5. Intubate patients who have increasing trouble breathing, increasing inability to clear secretions or protect airway, worsening FVC ($< 15\,mL/kg$), and worsening hypoxia.[4]
6. Nondepolarizing agents such as rocuronium (reduced dose $0.6\,mg/kg$) or vecuronium (reduced dose $0.08\,mg/kg$) are preferred paralytic agents, as lack of ACh receptors can make patients resistant to succinylcholine.[5]
7. Initial ventilator settings:
   - Mode of ventilation: assist control.
   - Initial FiO_2: 100%; once the patient stabilizes, titrate it down to maintain SpO_2 at 90%–94%.
   - PEEP: $5cmH_2O$.
   - Tidal volume (VT) 8–10 mL/kg of predicted (ideal) body weight:
     - Male: PBW (kg) = 50 + 2.3(height(in)-60)
     - Female: PBW (kg) = 45.5 + 2.3(height(in)-60)
   - RR: 12–16 breaths per minute; titrate to maintain normal pH of 7.35–7.45.
   - Inspiratory to expiratory (I/E) ratio of 1:3.
   - Maintain plateau pressure (Pplat) $\leq 30cmH_2O$ to avoid barotrauma.
   - Monitor clinical response, Pplat, and ABG closely.[5]
8. Once the airway is secured, investigate the causes of myasthenic crisis.
9. Initiate plasmapheresis (patient will need Hickman catheter placed) to remove circulating autoimmune antibodies, one plasma exchange every other day for five treatments, which will lead to improvement of symptoms in 2 days, with short-term benefit for 4 weeks.[6]
10. If plasmapheresis is not available or contraindicated, immunotherapy with IV gamma globulin $400\,mg/kg$ for 5 days will lead to improvement of symptoms in 4–5 days; more sustained efficacy for 4–8 weeks.[7]

References

1. Godoy DA, Mello LJ, Napoli MD. The myasthenic patient in crisis: an update of the management in Neurointensive Care Unit. *Arq Neuropsiquiatr.* 2013;71(9A):627–639.
2. Wu JY, Kuo PH, Fan PC, et al. The role of non-invasive ventilation and factors predicting extubation outcome in myasthenic crisis. *Neurocrit Care.* 2009;10:35–42.
3. Seneviratne J, Mandrekar J, Wijdicks EF, Rabinstein AA. Noninvasive ventilation in myasthenic crisis. *Arch Neurol.* 2008;65:54–58.
4. Adams J, Barton ED. *Emergency Medicine: Clinical Essentials.* Philadelphia: Elsevier Saunders; 2013.
5. Wendell LC, Levine JM. Myasthenic crisis. *Neurohospitalist.* 2011;1(1):16–22.
6. Saperstein DS, Barohn RJ. Management of myasthenia gravis. *Semin Neurol.* 2004;24(1):41–48.
7. Patwa HS, Chaudhry V, Katzberg H, Rae-Grant AD, So YT. Evidence-based guideline: intravenous immunoglobulins in the treatment of neuromuscular disorders: report of the Therapeutics and Technology Assessment Subcommittee of the American Academy of Neurology. *Neurolgy.* 2012;78(13):1009–1015.

Guillain-Barre Syndrome

Presentation

Guillain-Barre syndrome is an acute immune-mediated inflammatory demyelinating polyradiculoneuropathy with symmetric ascending muscular weakness and reduced deep tendon reflexes. GBS usually occurs 2–4 weeks after a respiratory or gastrointestinal illness. Infectious agents produce antibodies against gangliosides and glycolipids in the myelin of the peripheral nervous system. *Campylobacter jejuni* is the most commonly isolated infectious agent; however, other pathogens such as cytomegalovirus, Epstein-Barr virus, influenza virus, and varicella zoster virus have been reported.[1]

Initially, symptoms include finger and toe dysesthesia (painful, itchy, and burning fingers and toes) and symmetric calf and thigh muscle weakness that usually occur 2–4 weeks after respiratory or gastrointestinal illness. Muscular weakness will progress over hours to days to involve arms, trunk, cranial nerves (facial droop, ptosis, diplopia, pupillary abnormalities, dysarthria, dysphagia), and muscles of respiration, causing dyspnea. Patients may report pain in shoulders, back, buttocks, and thighs. Patients may also experience facial flushing, diaphoresis, constipation, diarrhea, and urinary retention as a result of autonomic dysfunction. On examination, patients may be tachypneic, with poor inspiratory effort, diminished breath sounds, hyporeflexia, or flaccid paralysis making them nonambulatory.[1]

Causes for Rapid Response Activation

Progressively worsening dyspnea, tachypnea, hypoxia, tachycardia, bradycardia, severe hypertension, hypotension.

Actions

INITIAL MEASURES

1. Continuous pulse oximetry.
2. Supplemental oxygen to maintain $SpO_2 > 92\%$ or $PaO_2 > 60–65\,mmHg$; transition to high flow oxygen when patient requires high flow rates.
3. Continuous cardiac monitoring.
4. Continuous capnography.
5. Transfer patients with labile dysautonomia, forced vital capacity (FVC) $< 20\,mL/kg$, severe bulbar palsy, and respiratory compromise to ICU.[2]

DIAGNOSTIC WORK-UP

1. Labs: CBC (leukocytosis in infection), CMP (concomitant electrolyte abnormalities, impaired renal function), CK, ESR, stool culture for *C. jejuni*, urine pregnancy test. Serum antibodies (anti-GM1 or anti-GQ1b antibodies) only in patients with questionable GBS.[2]

2. Needle electromyography (EMG) will demonstrate slow nerve conduction velocities, prolonged distal and F-wave latencies, conduction block, abnormal temporal dispersion, and other evidence of demyelination.[1,2]

3. Lumbar puncture: elevated protein > 400 mg/L without an elevation in white blood cells strongly supports the diagnosis.

TREATMENT

1. Suction pulmonary secretions.
2. Order chest physiotherapy.
3. One third of the patients will require intubation and mechanical ventilation[3]; therefore, frequent serial pulmonary function tests (PFTs) at bedside will help to monitor respiratory status.
4. Intubate if:
   - FVC (forced vital capacity) < 15 mL/kg (normal is 60–70 mL/kg)
   - NIF (negative inspiratory force) $\leq$ 30 cmH$_2$O (normal is > 60 cmH$_2$O)
   - Maximal inspiratory pressure < 30 cmH$_2$O
   - Maximal expiratory pressure < 40 cmH$_2$O
   - Reduction of more than 30% in vital capacity, maximal inspiratory pressure, or maximal expiratory pressure[4]
5. Initial ventilator settings:
   - Mode of ventilation: assist control.
   - Initial FiO$_2$: 100%; once the patient stabilizes, titrate it down to maintain SpO$_2$ at 90%–94%.
   - PEEP: 5 cmH$_2$O.
   - Tidal volume (VT) 8–10 mL/kg of predicted (ideal) body weight:
     - Male: PBW (kg) = 50 + 2.3(height(in)-60)
     - Female: PBW (kg) = 45.5 + 2.3(height(in)-60)
   - RR: 12–16 breaths per minute; titrate to maintain normal pH of 7.35–7.45.
   - Inspiratory to expiratory (I/E) ratio of 1:3.
   - Maintain plateau pressure (Pplat) $\leq$ 30 cmH$_2$O to avoid barotrauma.
   - Monitor clinical response, Pplat, and ABG closely.[5]
6. Identify and treat infection (UTI, pneumonia, bacteremia).
7. Due to autonomic instability, treat hypertension with short-acting antihypertensives such as:
   o Esmolol, with loading dose 500 µg/kg IV over 1 min, followed by 50 µg/kg/min; titrate to maximum of 200 µg/kg/min.[6]
   o Labetalol 20 mg IV bolus; may repeat doses of 20–80 mg IV at 10 min intervals until goal blood pressure achieved, with maximum 24 h total of 300 mg[6]; dose reduction may be needed in hepatic impairment.
8. Treat hypotension with supine position and IV fluids.
9. Both plasma exchange and IVIG decrease recovery time by 50% and have equal efficacy; combination of plasma exchange and IVIG does not shorten duration of illness and does not improve outcome.[1]
10. IV immunoglobulin (IVIG) 400 mg/kg bodyweight daily for 5 consecutive days is preferred treatment in many centers, as it is convenient, available, and is also preferred in hemodynamically unstable patients.[1]
11. Plasma exchange (patient will need Hickman catheter placed) to remove antibodies, most effective when started within 7 days of onset of illness; there are no available guidelines on volume of plasma removed and the optimal number of plasma exchange sessions;

however, many clinicians use North American protocol in which a total of 200–250 mL/ kg is exchanged over 7–10 days depending on the severity of the illness.[1]

References

1. Meena AK, et al. Treatment guidelines for Guillain-Barre syndrome. *Ann Indian Acad Neurol.* 2011;14(l1):S73–S81.
2. Andary MT, et al. *Guillain-Barre syndrome.* Emedicine.medscape.com. Updated: June 24, 2020.
3. Hughes RA, Wijdicks EF, Benson E, et al. Supportive care for patients with Guillain-Barré syndrome: Multidisciplinary Consensus Group. *Arch Neurol.* 2005;62:1194–1198.
4. Lawn ND, et al. Anticipating mechanical ventilation in Guillain-Barre syndrome. *Arch Neurol.* 2001;58(6):893–898.
5. Wendell LC, Levine JM. Myasthenic crisis. *Neurohospitalist.* 2011;1(1):16–22.
6. Levy ZD, Zhou Q, Slesinger TL. Hypertensive crises. *Critical Care Emergency Medicine.* 2nd ed. McGrawHill Education; vol. 17; 2017:175–183.

Serotonin Syndrome

Presentation

Serotonin syndrome occurs in patients taking selective serotonin reuptake inhibitors (SSRIs), most commonly with increase in prior prescription dosage or in combination with other medications. Less commonly, serotonin syndrome can happen in patients taking SSRIs at regular therapeutic doses. In hospital setting, serotonin syndrome can occur if other medications are added to SSRIs, such as ondansetron or metoclopramide to treat nausea, trazodone to treat insomnia, and opioids such as tramadol or fentanyl to treat pain.[1]

Symptoms include pressured speech, confusion, agitation, ataxia (lack of coordination, gait abnormalities), headache, heavy sweating, nausea, vomiting, diarrhea, goose bumps, twitching muscles, shivering, resting tremors, and myoclonic jerks. On examination, patients may have hyperthermia, tachycardia, elevated blood pressure, dilated pupils, clonus, or hyperreflexia.[2]

Causes for Rapid Response Activation

Severe agitation, tachycardia, severe hypertension, seizures, progressively worsening mental status changes, loss of consciousness.

Actions

1. Continuous pulse oximetry.
2. Supplemental oxygen to maintain $SpO_2 > 95\%$.
3. Continuous cardiac monitoring and blood pressure measurements.
4. Use Hunter Serotonin Toxicity Criteria (84% sensitivity) to assist with diagnosis.[1]
5. Discontinue all serotonergic medications.
6. Transfer patients to ICU if they are hyperthermic ($\geq 40°C$), have EKG evidence of dysrhythmias, or require vasopressors or intubation and mechanical ventilation.[2]
7. Consult poison control or toxicologist early in the course of rapid response.

DIAGNOSTIC WORK-UP

1. Labs: CBC, CMP, CK, magnesium, phosphorus, lactate, urine toxicology screen, serum salicylate, serum acetaminophen, and coagulation studies (PT/aPTT/INR) to assess for DIC, blood cultures if febrile; generally, labs are done to exclude other conditions.
2. Order EKG to assess for QT prolongation.
3. Order head CT scan in stable patients with new onset seizure, focal neurological findings, or hypertension.
4. Order lumbar puncture in febrile patients.

TREATMENT

1. Treat dehydration, hypotension, and rhabdomyolysis with IV fluids.
2. Due to autonomic instability, treat hypertension with short-acting antihypertensives such as:

o Esmolol, with loading dose 500 µg/kg IV over 1 min, followed by 50 µg/kg/min; titrate to maximum of 200 µg/kg/min.[3]

o Labetalol 20 mg IV bolus; may repeat doses of 20–80 mg IV at 10 min intervals until goal blood pressure achieved, with maximum 24 h total of 300 mg[3]; dose reduction might be needed in hepatic impairment.

3. Treat hyperthermia with cooling blankets, cool sponging, fans, and cold saline[4] to prevent DIC or multiorgan failure.

4. Treat agitation and tremors with benzodiazepines.

5. Intubation and mechanical ventilation is indicated in patients unable to protect their airway, with rapid decline in respiratory status, with severe muscle rigidity, or with worsening hyperthermia with temperature > 41°C; avoid succinylcholine as a paralytic in rhabdomyolysis to prevent hyperkalemia; use rocuronium or vecuronium instead.[2]

6. Treat moderate-to-severe serotonin syndrome with cyproheptadine (5HT antagonist) 4 mg po every hour for three doses, followed by 4–8 mg po every 6 h as needed to control symptoms; maximum dose is 20 mg/day; it is available only in oral form; crush and administer via NG tube in altered patients unable to have PO intake; in elderly patients, use reduced dose of 4 mg every 12 h.[5]

References

1. Ables AZ, Nagubilli R. Prevention, diagnosis and management of serotonin syndrome. *Am Fam Physician.* 2010;81(9):1139–1142.

2. Cushing TA, et al. *Selective Serotonin Reuptake Inhibitor Toxicity.* Emedicine.medscape.com. Updated: April 24, 2018.

3. Levy ZD, Zhou Q, Slesinger TL. Hypertensive crises. *Critical Care. Emergency Medicine.* 2nd ed. McGrawHill Education; vol. 17; 2017:175–183.

4. Wasserman DD, et al. *Cooling Techniques for Hyperthermia.* StatPearls Publishing; 2020. ncbi.nlm.nih.gov.

5. *Cyproheptadine.* Reference.medscape.com.

Neuroleptic Malignant Syndrome

Presentation

Neuroleptic malignant syndrome is a rare life-threatening idiosyncratic reaction to dopamine receptor antagonists, such as neuroleptic medications. It may happen within 4–14 days (usually 10 days) after initiation of neuroleptic medication or after increase in dose.[1]

Neuroleptic medications are antipsychotic medications, including typical antipsychotics such as haloperidol or atypical antipsychotics such as quetiapine, olanzapine, and risperidone, among others. Other medications that can cause neuroleptic malignant syndrome include metoclopramide, promethazine, among others. Abrupt discontinuation of dopaminergic medications, such as anti-Parkinson medications, such as levodopa, bromocriptine, or amantadine, can also cause neuroleptic malignant syndrome.[1]

Symptoms include hyperthermia (temperature $> 38°C$), dysphagia, dystonia, dyskinesia, resting tremor, shuffling gait, muscular rigidity, altered mental status, and autonomic dysfunction such as skin pallor, diaphoresis, sialorrhea (excessive salivation), flushing, and urinary incontinence.[2]

Muscle rigidity is a very important symptom of neuroleptic malignant syndrome and can cause muscle damage; therefore, patients will have laboratory changes such as hyperkalemia, elevated liver function tests, elevated creatinine kinase, and elevated LDH. Patients are at high risk of severe rhabdomyolysis development.[2]

Causes for Rapid Response Activation

Tachycardia, progressively worsening tachypnea, dyspnea, hypoxia, lethargy, psychomotor agitation.

Actions

INITIAL MEASURES

1. Continuous pulse oximetry.
2. Supplemental oxygen to maintain $SpO_2 > 95\%$.
3. Continuous cardiac and blood pressure monitoring.
4. Discontinue all neuroleptic agents.
5. If the syndrome occurred due to abrupt discontinuation of dopaminergic medication, the medication should be restarted as soon as possible.
6. Transfer the patient to ICU.
7. Consult neurologist early in the course of rapid response.
8. Consult psychiatrist to assist with management of the underlying psychiatric illness in the setting of discontinued neuroleptics.

DIAGNOSTIC WORK-UP

1. Order ABG in patients with respiratory distress.

2. Labs: CBC (leukocytosis, thrombocytosis), CMP (hyperkalemia, metabolic acidosis, hypocalcemia, elevated AST, ALT, alkaline phosphatase), LDH (elevated), CK (elevated), uric acid (elevated), serum iron (decreased), phosphate (elevated), urinalysis (proteinuria), urine myoglobin level, coagulation studies, urine toxicology screen, serum salicylate, and serum acetaminophen.
3. Order chest X-ray to assess for pneumonia, pleural effusions, atelectasis, or pulmonary vascular congestion.
4. Obtain CT scan or MRI of the brain to exclude other conditions, such as intracranial hemorrhage or structural lesions.
5. Order lumbar puncture to exclude meningitis in patients with fever and altered mental status.

TREATMENT

1. Treat hyperthermia with antipyretics, cooling blankets, cool sponging, fans, and cold saline.[3]
2. Treat dehydration, hypotension, rhabdomyolysis, acute kidney injury with IV fluid resuscitation.
3. Treat agitation with benzodiazepines.
4. Start intubation and mechanical ventilation for patients unable to protect their airway due to excessive salivation, dysphagia, or coma; patients with worsening respiratory status; and patients with severe hyperthermia or muscle rigidity.
5. Administer sodium bicarbonate 50–150 mEq diluted in 1 L of D5W at a rate of 100–200 mL/h IV in patients with rhabdomyolysis to alkalinize urine and prevent renal failure; continue drip until correction of urine pH to 6–8.[4]
6. The following medications can be administered alone or in combination; however, their use is controversial:
   o Dantrolene (inhibits calcium release from a sarcoplasmic reticulum); start with initial bolus of 1–2.5 mg/kg, followed by 1 mg/kg every 6 h, with maximum dose of 10 mg/kg/day (has risk of hepatotoxicity).[2]
   o Bromocriptine (dopamine agonist) orally or via nasogastric tube; start at 2.5 mg two or three times daily and increase the dose by 2.5 mg every 24 h until response is achieved, with maximum dose of 45 mg/day.[2]

References

1. Benzer TI. *Neuroleptic Malignant Syndrome.* Emedicine.medscape.com. Updated: December 07, 2020.
2. Berman BD. Neuroleptic malignant syndrome. *Neurohospitalist.* 2011;1(1):41–47.
3. Wasserman DD, et al. *Cooling Techniques for Hyperthermia.* StatPearls Publishing; 2020. ncbi.nlm.nih.gov.
4. *Sodium bicarbonate.* Drugs/com.

CHAPTER 4

Gastrointestinal Emergencies

Upper Gastrointestinal Bleeding

Presentation

Upper GI bleeding includes bleeding from the esophagus to the ligament of Treitz. Causes of upper GI bleeding include peptic ulcer disease, esophageal and gastric varices, AVM (arteriovenous malformations), esophagitis, gastritis, duodenitis, Mallory-Weiss tear, or malignancy.

Nonvariceal upper GI bleeding is associated with nonsteroidal antiinflammatory drug (NSAIDs) use, aspirin, clopidogrel, warfarin, direct-acting oral anticoagulants, SSRIs, corticosteroids, and *Helicobacter pylori* infection. Variceal upper GI bleeding is associated with liver cirrhosis/portal hypertension.

Patients with upper GI bleeding may present with dyspepsia, heartburn, chest pain, epigastric pain, coffee-ground-like emesis, hematemesis (vomiting of blood), and melena (black tarry sticky stools). On examination, patients may have upper epigastric tenderness or guarding.

Causes for Rapid Response Activation

Tachycardia, hypotension, worsening altered mental status (confusion, anxiety), syncope.

Actions

INITIAL MEASURES

1. Maintain continuous pulse oximetry
2. Administer supplemental oxygen to maintain $SpO_2 > 92\%$
3. Continuous cardiac and blood pressure monitoring
4. Hold all NSAIDs, anticoagulants, and antiplatelets
5. Order NPO
6. Consult gastroenterologist early in the course of rapid response
7. Transfer patients with anticipated hemodynamic instability, especially elderly patients with comorbidities, to ICU
8. Insert two large-bore IV catheters (16 gauge or larger) into peripheral veins; place central venous line if peripheral access cannot be established[1]

DIAGNOSTIC WORK-UP

1. Labs: Type and crossmatch blood (for 2–6 units depending on the severity of bleeding), CBC (need hemoglobin level every 4–6 h, platelet count), BMP (blood in upper intestine elevates BUN; BUN/creatinine ratio > 36 in a patient without renal insufficiency is

suggestive of upper GI bleed; monitor calcium level in patients receiving multiple blood transfusions), PT/aPTT/INR, gastrin (to identify rare patients with gastrinoma, especially for patients with multiple ulcers), and stool occult blood test.

2. Order EKG in patients with serious cardiac disease.
3. Order CT scan abdomen/pelvis in patients with high suspicion of unusual causes of upper GI bleed, such as pancreatitis with pseudocyst hemorrhage, hemorrhagic cholecystitis, or aorto-enteric fistula (e.g., patients with h/o pancreaticobiliary procedure or aortic reconstruction).[2]

TREATMENT

1. Start volume resuscitation: 20 mL/kg bolus of crystalloid; repeat until resolution of tachycardia and hypotension.[1]
2. Transfuse pRBC in all patients with evidence of hemorrhagic shock (HR > 100 and SBP < 100) regardless of the level of Hg; in hemodynamically stabilized patients, transfuse if Hg < 7; in cardiac disease, transfuse if Hg < 8.[3]
3. If INR > 1.5, transfuse FFP 4–6 units; consider vitamin K 10 mg IV in life-threatening bleeding; as effect of vitamin K may last 1–2 weeks, reversal with vitamin K should be weighed against the future need to chronically anticoagulate the patient.[1,4]
4. If platelets < 50,000/mm,[3] transfuse platelets.[4]
5. Administer pantoprazole 80 mg IV bolus, followed by 8 mg/h drip[5] for up to 72 h, at which point transition to high-dose oral PPI.
6. For variceal upper GI bleed, add:
   ■ Octreotide 50 μg bolus, followed by 25–50 μg/h infusion for 3–5 days[6]; use is controversial
   ■ Ceftriaxone 1 g IV daily or ciprofloxacin 500 mg IV every 12 h[6] to reduce overall mortality and risk of re-bleeding
7. EGD should be done within 12 h after arrival to ER for clip placement + epinephrine injection or cauterization + epinephrine injection for ulcers with active bleeding, non-bleeding visible vessels and adherent clot with an underlying vessel visualized after clot removal,[5] and variceal ligation for variceal bleeding.
8. Obtain CT angiography (CTA) of abdomen/pelvis if bleeding persists despite medical/endoscopic treatment or if bleeding persists in the setting of negative endoscopy, followed by interventional radiology consultation for transcatheter arterial embolization (TAE).
9. If patient with variceal upper GI bleed failed medical and endoscopic therapy, consult interventional radiology for TIPS (transjugular intrahepatic portosystemic shunt).[4]
10. If patient has severe life-threatening hemorrhage that is persistent and not responsive to above resuscitation, consult general surgery for operative management of probable perforated viscus.

References

1. Elie-Turenne MC, Hwang CW, Zeglam TM. Gastrointestinal bleeding. *Critical Care. Emergency Medicine.* 2nd ed. McGrawHill Education; 2017;23:241–259.
2. Frattaroli FM, Casciani E, Spoletini D, et al. Prospective study comparing multidetector row CT and endoscopy in acute gastrointestinal bleeding. *World J Surg.* 2009;33(10):2209–2217.
3. Villanueva C. Transfusion strategies for acute upper gastrointestinal bleeding. *N Engl J Med.* 2013;368:11–21.
4. Barnert J. Diagnosis and management of lower gastrointestinal bleeding. *Nat Rev Gastroenterol Hepatol.* 2009;6:637–646.
5. Arbo JE, Ruoss S, et al. Gastrointestinal hemorrhage. *Decision-Making in Emergency Critical Care. An Evidence-Based Handbook*; 2015;24:324–333.
6. Garcia-Tsao G. Prevention and management of gastroesophageal varices and variceal hemorrhage in cirrhosis. *Am J Gastroenterol.* 2007;102:2086–2102.

Lower Gastrointestinal Bleeding

Presentation

Lower gastrointestinal bleeding occurs from a source distal to the ileocecal valve,[1] such as colon, rectum, or anus. Causes of lower GI bleeding include diverticular hemorrhage (most common cause), internal hemorrhoids, ischemic colitis, inflammatory bowel disease, recent colonoscopy with polypectomy (postpolypectomy bleeding), colorectal cancer, vascular ectasia, prior abdominal and/or pelvic radiation (e.g., for prostate malignancy), prior surgery (anastomotic bleeding), and abdominal aortic aneurysm with aorto-enteric fistula.[2]

Older age and medications such as nonsteroidal antiinflammatory drugs (NSAID), aspirin, clopidogrel, warfarin, and direct-acting oral anticoagulants increase the risk for lower GI bleeding.

Patients may present with abdominal cramps, melena (black tarry sticky stools) from cecal source, hematochezia such as maroon stools from right colon source or BRBPR (bright red blood per rectum) from left colon source. Clinical factors predictive of severe colonic bleeding include aspirin use, at least two comorbid illnesses, heart rate > 100/min, and systolic blood pressure < 115 mmHg.[3]

Causes for Rapid Response Activation

Tachycardia, hypotension, progressively worsening altered mental status such as confusion and lethargy, syncope.

Actions

INITIAL MEASURES

1. Maintain continuous pulse oximetry
2. Administer supplemental oxygen to maintain $SpO_2 > 92\%$
3. Maintain continuous cardiac monitoring/blood pressure measurements/orthostatics with caution
4. Consult gastroenterologist early in the course of rapid response
5. Transfer to ICU hemodynamically unstable patients, patients with persistent active bleeding and underlying bleeding disorders, patients with serios comorbidities, and elderly patients
6. Order NPO
7. Hold all NSAIDs, anticoagulants, and antiplatelets
8. Insert two large-bore IV catheters (16 gauge or larger) into peripheral veins; place central venous line if peripheral access cannot be established[4]
9. Type and crossmatch blood (for 2–6 units depending on the severity of the bleeding)

DIAGNOSTIC WORK-UP

1. Labs: CBC (need hemoglobin level every 4–6 h), BMP (monitor calcium level in patients receiving multiple blood transfusions), and coagulation studies (PT/INR/aPTT).
2. Order EKG in patients with serious cardiac disease.
3. Order plain abdominal radiography if there is any suspicion of perforation or obstruction, as these would be contraindications for colonoscopy.

TREATMENT

1. Start volume resuscitation with 20 mL/kg bolus of crystalloid; repeat until resolution of tachycardia and hypotension[4]; the goal is normalization of vital signs before endoscopic intervention.
2. Transfuse pRBC in all patients with evidence of hemorrhagic shock (HR > 100 and SBP < 100) regardless of the level of Hg. In hemodynamically stabilized patients, transfuse if Hg < 7; in cardiac disease, transfuse if Hg < 8.[3]
3. If INR > 1.5, transfuse FFP.[5]
4. If platelets < 50,000/mm[3], transfuse platelets.[5]
5. In massive transfusion (transfusion of > 10 units of pRBC within 24 h), transfuse platelets and FFP in a ratio of one unit of platelets and fresh frozen plasma per unit of RBCs transfused.[6]
6. Severe hematochezia with hemodynamic instability could be indicative of brisk upper GI bleeding, especially in patients taking antiplatelets and/or anticoagulants, in patients with a history of peptic ulcer disease, or patients with liver cirrhosis with portal hypertension; severe hematochezia should be assessed with upper endoscopy.
7. Colonoscopy is the initial diagnostic procedure recommended for patients with lower GI bleeding and will identify the bleeding site in 48%–90% of patients; unprepped colonoscopy or sigmoidoscopy is not recommended.[6]
8. In hemodynamically stable patients without obstruction/perforation and with ongoing bleeding, start rapid bowel purge prep with 4–6 L of GoLYTELY, to be administered as 1 L orally every 30–45 min,[6] followed by colonoscopy within 24 h.
9. If patient is unable to tolerate rapid drinking of GoLYTELY, place NG tube to administer GoLYTELY.[6]
10. Consider administration of prokinetic agent such as metoclopramide 10 mg IV immediately before starting colon prep to reduce nausea and improve gastric emptying.[6]
11. Emergent unprepped hydroflush colonoscopy is reserved for hemodynamically stable patients with large amount of blood in GI tract; blood will act as a cathartic and clean the GI tract from stool; these patients can be treated with 1 L of tap water enemas three to four times over 1 h prior to colonoscopy; during the colonoscopy, gastroenterologist will use a hydro-jet irrigation with a high-powered mechanical suction system to facilitate removal of adherent residual stool.[6]
12. Endoscopic therapy should be provided to patients with high-risk stigmata, such as active bleeding (spurting or oozing), nonbleeding visible vessel, or adherent clot:
    - Diverticular bleeding: clips
    - Angioectasia: argon plasma coagulation
    - Postpolypectomy bleeding: clip or contact thermal therapy with or without epinephrine injection[6]
13. In obscure lower GI bleeding when colonoscopy failed to identify the site of bleeding, proceed with CT angiography (CTA) and consult interventional radiologist for visceral angiography with embolization with coil springs, Gelfoam, polyvinyl alcohol, or oxidized cellulose.

14. In hemodynamically unstable patients with massive ongoing lower GI bleeding, consult interventional radiologist for visceral angiography with embolization.

15. Consult general surgeon for laparotomy/segmental bowel resection for patients with persistent bleeding refractory to medical/endoscopic/embolization treatment or colonic tumors; patients who are actively bleeding from an unknown source will need subtotal colectomy.

References

1. Raju GS, Gerson L, Das A, et al. American Gastroenterological Association Institute technical review on obscure gastrointestinal bleeding. *Gastroenterology.* 2007;133:1697–1717.

2. Ghassemi KA, Jensen DM. Lowe GI bleeding: epidemiology and management. *Curr Gastroenterol Rep.* 2013;15(7):10.

3. Strate LL, et al. Early predictors of severity in acute lower intestinal tract bleeding. *Arch Intern Med.* 2003;163(7):838–843.

4. Elie-Turenne MC, Hwang CW, Zeglam TM. Gastrointestinal bleeding. *Critical Care. Emergency Medicine.* 2nd ed. McGrawHill Education; vol. 23; 2017:241–259.

5. Villanueva C. Transfusion strategies for acute upper gastrointestinal bleeding. *N Engl J Med.* 2013;368:11–21.

6. Strate LL, Gralnek IM. ACG clinical guideline: management of patients with acute lower gastrointestinal bleeding. *Am J Gastroenterol.* 2016;111(4):459–474.

Acute Liver Failure

Presentation

Acute liver failure is a rare condition characterized by rapid decline of liver function resulting in coagulopathy (INR ≥ 1.5) and encephalopathy in the absence of preexisting liver disease.[1] It is associated with high mortality.

Causes of acute liver failure include acetaminophen toxicity; idiosyncratic drug reactions (e.g., amoxicillin-clavulanate, ciprofloxacin, amiodarone, labetalol, statins, phenytoin, valproic acid); shock; hepatitis A, B, E; hepatitis caused by HSV; cytomegalovirus or Epstein Barr virus; hepatic vein thrombosis (Budd-Chiari syndrome); portal vein thrombosis, Wilson disease; autoimmune hepatitis; or exposure to hepatic toxins such as mushrooms (Amanita phalloides), phosphorus in fireworks, or organic solvents.[1] Acetaminophen poisoning is the leading cause of acute liver failure in the United States.[1] Acute liver failure is usually associated with ingestion of $> 10\,g$ of acetaminophen.[1]

Common symptoms are fatigue, nausea, vomiting, diarrhea, and jaundice; scleral icterus; right upper quadrant pain; ascites; altered mental status (encephalopathy) such as irritability, confusion, or lethargy; and increased intracranial pressure due to cerebral edema.[1]

Grades of Hepatic Encephalopathy[2]

Grade 0—Subclinical, normal mental status, but minimal changes in memory, concentration, cognitive function, and coordination

Grade 1—Mild confusion, euphoria or depression, decreased attention, slowing of ability to perform mental tasks, irritability, disorder of sleep pattern

Grade 2—Drowsiness, lethargy, gross deficits in ability to perform mental tasks, obvious personality changes, inappropriate behavior, intermittent disorientation (usually with regard to time)

Grade 3—Somnolent, but arousable state, inability to perform mental tasks, disorientation with regard to time and place, marked confusion, amnesia, occasional fits of rage, speech present but incomprehensible

Grade 4—Coma, with or without response to painful stimuli

Causes for Rapid Response Activation

Rapid response may be called due to signs of elevated intracranial pressure related to cerebral edema, such as worsening altered mental status, hypertension and bradycardia, or hypotension and tachycardia.

Actions

INITIAL MEASURES

1. Maintain continuous pulse oximetry
2. Administer supplemental oxygen to maintain $SpO_2 > 92\%$

3. Maintain continuous cardiac monitoring/blood pressure measurements
4. Patients will likely be better managed in a tertiary care hospital with liver transplantation capability
5. Order NPO
6. Determine the stage of encephalopathy[2]
7. Use MELD (model for end-stage liver disease) score for prognosis; MELD score > 30.5 predicts a need for liver transplantation[3]

DIAGNOSTIC WORK-UP

1. Order ABG to assess severity of hypoxia.
2. Labs: CBC (thrombocytopenia), BMP (electrolytes, renal function, hypoglycemia), liver function tests (elevated), PT/INR/aPTT (severity of coagulopathy), serum ammonia (elevated), lactate (elevated), phosphate, magnesium, acetaminophen level in patients with acetaminophen toxicity; if Wilson disease is highly suspected, consider serum free copper and ceruloplasmin levels (low)[3]; check viral serologies for hepatitis A, B and, if patient is pregnant, hepatitis E[3]; check autoimmune markers such as ANA (antinuclear antibody) and ASMA (antismooth muscle antibody)[3]; check HSV serologies/DNA[3]; and do urine pregnancy test in female patients of child-bearing age.
3. Order a Doppler ultrasonography scan of the liver to assess ascites, size and texture of the liver, patency and flow in the hepatic veins (Budd-Chiari syndrome), the hepatic artery and the portal vein, liver masses, or to exclude biliary tract obstruction.[1]
4. Order CT scan of abdomen without contrast to assess other intra-abdominal pathology.
5. Order CT scan of head without contrast to exclude intracranial hemorrhage, especially in patients with stage III or IV encephalopathy and also after the insertion or removal of ICP monitor to check positioning and hemorrhage.[1]
6. Order electroencephalography (EEG) in patients with suspicion of subtle or nonconvulsive seizures.

TREATMENT

1. Patients may need IV glucose, such as a 10% dextrose solution, to prevent hypoglycemia.
2. Start volume resuscitation in hypotensive patients with 20–25 mL/kg of isotonic crystalloid.[1]
3. If patient is refractory to initial fluid challenge, start norepinephrine drip[4]:
   - Norepinephrine at 8–12 µg/min, with maintenance dose of 2–4 µg/min[5]
4. Replace electrolytes, such as phosphate, magnesium, and potassium.
5. Administer N-acetyl-cysteine (NAC) in acetaminophen toxicity, with loading dose of 150 mg/kg IV over 1 h, followed by 50 mg/kg over 4 h, then 100 mg/kg over 16 h; total dose is 300 mg/kg over 21 h; continue until INR < 1.5; most effective if administered within first 12 h after ingestion.[6]
6. Specific therapies should be discussed with transplantation team prior to initiation:
   - High dose IV penicillin G in mushroom poisoning (unproven efficacy)
   - Antiviral therapy (e.g., lamivudine or entecavir) in hepatitis B (unproven efficacy)
   - Antiviral therapy (e.g., acyclovir) in HSV hepatitis (unproven efficacy)
   - IV steroids in autoimmune hepatitis (unproven efficacy)
   - Chelation of copper and/or plasmapheresis in Wilson disease (unproven efficacy)
   - TIPS (transjugular intrahepatic portosystemic shunt) in Budd-Chiari syndrome
7. In patients with symptoms of intracranial hypertension:
   - Transfer to ICU patients with grade II encephalopathy.

- Elevate head of bed to 30° angle.
- Avoid movements increasing intracranial pressure, such as Valsalva maneuver, straining, coughing, or ventilator dyssynchrony.
- Control pain and agitation with fentanyl and propofol, respectively.
- Control fever with antipyretics such as rectal acetaminophen and cooling blankets.
- Consult with neurosurgery regarding ventricular catheter placement through a burr hole to monitor ICP; in patients with grade II–IV encephalopathy, this is needed to prevent brain herniation and to prolong survival while awaiting donor liver or survival of patient's own hepatocytes; goal ICP < 20 mmHg.
- Adequate reversal of coagulopathy should be achieved prior to placement of ICP monitor:
  - INR < 1.5
  - Platelets > 50,000 mm^3
  - Fibrinogen > 100 mg/dL
  - Normal PTT
- Hyperventilation causes decrease in pCO$_2$ with subsequent cerebral arteriolar constriction and reduced cerebral blood volume, which leads to decrease in ICP; effect lasts for < 24 h, and prolonged hyperventilation should be avoided.
- Administer mannitol as an initial bolus of 0.25–1 g/kg IV; this can be repeated at 0.25–0.5 g/kg IV doses every 6–8 h as needed. Renal toxicity is one of the primary concerns; therefore, check serum osmolarity to calculate osmolar gap (osmolar gap = measured serum osmolarity – calculated serum osmolarity); goal osmolar gap is < 18–20; other concerns include extravasation and fluid-electrolyte imbalance.
- If mannitol causes volume overload in patients with renal impairment, consult nephrologist to start hemodialysis to remove excess fluid.[1]

8. In patients with grade III encephalopathy:
   - Administer propofol 50 µg/kg/min before intubation; this is a sedative of choice as it reduces intracranial pressure; etomidate can also be used.
   - Start intubation and mechanical ventilation.
   - Use endotracheal lidocaine before endotracheal suctioning to avoid laryngeal stimulation-related spikes in ICP.
   - Place NG tube for decompression of stomach.[1]

9. In coagulopathy:
   - Administer four-factor PCC (Kcentra) or FFP if bleeding, or if not bleeding and INR > 7, or if invasive procedure (e.g., liver biopsy or ICP monitor placement) is planned, and vitamin K 10 mg IV.
   - If nonresponsive to FFP, consider recombinant factor VIIA (rFVIIA) 40 µg/kg IV; PT will normalize in 20 min and remain normal for 3–4 h; potential risk of DIC/arterial thrombotic events.
   - Administer platelets 6–8 units if platelet count is < 20,000 mm^3 or if invasive procedure is planned and platelet count is < 50,000 mm^3; this will increase platelet count to > 50,000 mm^3; transfused platelets may survive for 3–5 days.
   - Administer cryoprecipitate if fibrinogen < 100 mg/dL.[1,4]

10. Treat seizure with phenytoin 20 mg/kg IV; limit benzodiazepines due to delayed clearance of benzodiazepines by liver.

11. Consider empirical antibiotics such as piperacillin-tazobactam/fluconazole IV in patients listed for liver transplant who developed SIRS (systemic inflammatory response syndrome), refractory hypotension, and progression of hepatic encephalopathy to advanced stages.[4]

12. NPO patients may require TPN (with protein restriction) if enteral feeds are contraindicated.

13. Patients with acute kidney injury (AKI) may require dialysis; CVVHD (continuous venovenous hemodialysis) is preferred over intermittent hemodialysis, as it causes fewer fluid shifts.[1]

14. Liver biopsy may be considered when the cause of acute liver failure is unknown, or to confirm drug-induced liver injury or autoimmune hepatitis, or when immunosuppressive agents are being considered.

15. Liver transplantation is the definitive treatment of acute liver failure, or bioartificial liver when liver donor is not available.

References

1. Hsu CH, Menne AR, Tisherman SA. Acute liver failure. In: *Critical care Emergency Medicine*; 2017:261–272. [Chapter 24].

2. *What Is West Haven Classification System for Hepatic Encephalopathy?* . Emedicine.medscape.com.

3. Flamm SL, Yang Y, Singh S, et al. American Gastroenterological Association Institute guidelines for the diagnosis and management of acute liver failure. *Gastroenterology.* 2017;152(3):644–647.

4. Stravitz RT, Kramer AH, Davern T, et al. Intensive care of patients with acute liver failure: recommendations of the US Acute Liver Failure Study Group. *Crit Care Med.* 2007;35(11):2498–2508.

5. *Norepinephrine Dosage.* Drugs.com.

6. *Acetaminophen Dosage.* Drugs.com.

Severe Acute Pancreatitis

Presentation

Acute pancreatitis is a reversible inflammation of the pancreas. The most common causes of acute pancreatitis are gallstones and alcohol (80% of cases)[1]; other causes include drug reactions, recent invasive procedure, or hypertriglyceridemia. The diagnosis requires two of the following factors: abdominal pain, elevation of amylase or lipase > 3 times the upper limit of normal, or evidence of acute pancreatitis on imaging.[2] Symptoms may include anorexia, nausea, vomiting, upper abdominal pain, or diarrhea.

About 20% of patients with acute pancreatitis may develop severe degree, which is associated with 15% mortality.[3] Acute severe pancreatitis is defined by evidence of persistent (> 48 h) organ failure. Examples of acute organ failure include systolic blood pressure < 90 mmHg, $P_aO_2 \leq 60$ mmHg, serum creatinine level ≥ 2 mg/dL, or GI bleeding amounting to ≥ 500 mL/24 h. Acute organ failure can happen in complications such as abscess, necrosis, or pseudocyst.

Causes for Rapid Response Activation

Progressively worsening dyspnea, tachycardia, hypotension, hematemesis, melena, listlessness.

Actions

INITIAL MEASURES

1. Maintain continuous pulse oximetry
2. Administer supplemental oxygen to maintain $SpO_2 > 92\%$
3. Maintain continuous cardiac monitoring/blood pressure measurements
4. Order NPO/bowel rest
5. BISAP (bedside index of severity of acute pancreatitis) score is a simplified score that can be easily applied at patient's bedside in the early phase[4]:
   - BUN > 25 mg/dL
   - Impaired mental status
   - SIRS
   - Age > 60 years
   - Pleural effusion

   A BISAP score ≥ 2 is a statistically significant cutoff value for the diagnosis of severe acute pancreatitis, organ failure, and mortality[5]
6. Transfer to ICU patients with persistent organ dysfunction or failure despite adequate fluid resuscitation

DIAGNOSTIC WORK-UP

1. Order ABG in critically ill patients, to assess severity of hypoxia.
2. Labs: CBC (hematocrit > 44% is an independent risk factor of pancreatic necrosis), CMP (BUN > 20 mg/dL is an independent predictor of mortality), lipase (more specific and

reliable than amylase), triglyceride level (> 1000 mg/dL is diagnostic of pancreatitis due to hypertriglyceridemia), CRP (> 15 mg/L is used as a prognostic factor), and procalcitonin (≥ 3.8 ng/mL is predictive of infected necrosis of pancreas).[5]

3. Perform an upright KUB (kidneys, ureters, bladder) to assess the presence of free air in abdomen.
4. Order contrast-enhanced CT scan of abdomen and pelvis to assess extension of pancreatic or peripancreatic necrosis; the scan will also be useful to assess mesenteric ischemia; however, an early CT scan will miss necrosis; 90%–100% sensitivity may occur 4 days after necrosis.[6]
5. MRI can be considered in patients with iodinated contrast allergy or patients with chronic kidney disease.
6. Order MRCP (magnetic resonance cholangiopancreatography) or EUS (endoscopic ultrasound) to screen for occult common bile duct stones (choledocholithiasis) in patients with unknown etiology.

TREATMENT

1. Start goal-directed IVF resuscitation, such as NS or LR 20 mL/kg for 60–90 min, followed by 250–500 mL/h for the next 48 h to maintain urine output of 0.5 mL/kg/h, except in patients with cardiovascular and renal comorbidities; frequently reassess fluid status[7]; avoid overresuscitation to prevent abdominal compartment syndrome.
2. For pain control, may consider PCA; hydromorphone (Dilaudid) is preferred over morphine or fentanyl in nonintubated patients; consider epidural analgesia for patients requiring high dose of opioids for extended period of time.[5]
3. Prophylactic antibiotics are no longer recommended, even in patients with acute severe pancreatitis, as they are not associated with significant decrease in morbidity or mortality.[1,5]
4. If you suspect infected acute pancreatitis (procalcitonin may be predictive of the risk of infected acute pancreatitis), consult interventional radiologist for CT-guided fine needle aspiration (FNA) of the necrotic focus and send collected fluid for Gram stain and cultures to guide antibiotic treatment.[5]
5. In patients with infected necrosis, empiric antibiotics should cover both aerobic and anaerobic Gram-positive and Gram-negative bacteria[5]; drug of choice is imipenem/cilastatin (Primaxin) 500 mg IV q6h[8]; other antibiotics that could be considered include:
   - Piperacillin/tazobactam (Zosyn) 3.375 g IV q6h[9]
   - Ticarcillin/clavulanate (Timentin) 3.1 g IV q4-6h[10]
   - Ceftazidime 2 g IV q8h[11]
   - Cefuroxime (Ceftin) 1.5 g IV q8h[12]
6. For patients with acute pancreatitis caused by hypertriglyceridemia, the following treatment is recommended:
   - Use regular insulin at 0.1–0.3 units/kg/h and 5% or 10% dextrose in water infusion at 150–200 mL/h, with close q1h glucose monitoring.
   - Heparin 5000 U SC q8h may be considered.
   - Plasmapheresis is reserved for patients with severe acute pancreatitis; patient will need placement of hemodialysis catheter.
   - Goal is to reduce triglycerides to < 500 mg/dL, at which time both insulin infusion and plasmapheresis can be stopped.
   - When patient is able to have oral intake, start first choice drug for treatment of hypertriglyceridemia—fibrate (fenofibrate 160 mg/day, gemfibrozil 600 mg po twice daily); other antilipemic drugs include niacin or statins.[13]
7. In patients with acute gallstone pancreatitis and no cholangitis, urgent ERCP is not recommended.[1,5]

8. In patients with acute gallstone pancreatitis and cholangitis or common bile duct obstruction, ERCP is recommended.[5]

9. In patients with severe acute gallstone pancreatitis, guidelines on ERCP are controversial.[5]

10. Percutaneous or endoscopic drainage is reserved for clinically deteriorating patients with infected necrotizing pancreatitis, such as ongoing organ failure, gastric outlet, biliary, or intestinal obstruction due to a large walled off necrosis (usually occurs 4 weeks after the onset of the disease), disconnected duct syndrome, or symptomatic or growing pseudocyst.[5]

11. Surgical interventions are reserved for the following cases:
    ▪ Refractory to percutaneous/endoscopic interventions
    ▪ Abdominal compartment syndrome
    ▪ Bowel ischemia
    ▪ Acute necrotizing cholecystitis
    ▪ Bowel fistula extending into a peripancreatic collection[5]

12. In patients with acute gallstone pancreatitis, cholecystectomy is recommended during the initial admission rather than after discharge.[1,5]

13. In patients with acute gallstone necrotizing pancreatitis, cholecystectomy should not be performed until acute inflammation has decreased (pain is resolving and lipase is trending down) and fluid collections are decreasing in size.

14. Start intubation and mechanical ventilation ventilation for patients in whom oxygen supply is not efficient for correction of tachypnea/dyspnea.[5]

References

1. Crockett SD, Wani S, Gardner TB, et al. American Gastroenterological Association Institute guideline on initial management of acute pancreatitis. *Gastroenterology.* 2018;154(4):1096–1101.

2. Banks PA, Bollen TL, Dervenis C, et al. Classification of acute pancreatitis – 2012; revision of the Atlanta classification and definitions by international consensus. *Gut.* 2013;62:102–111.

3. Van Santvoort HC, Bakker OJ, Bollen TL, et al. A conservative and minimally invasive approach to necrotizing pancreatitis improves outcome. *Gastroenterology.* 2011;141:1254–1263.

4. Wu BU, Johannes RS, Sun X, Tabak Y, Conwell DL, Banks PA. The early prediction of mortality in acute pancreatitis: a large population-based study. *Gut.* 2008;57:1698–1703.

5. Leppaniemi A, Tolonen M, Tarasconi A, et al. 2019 WSES guidelines for the management of severe acute pancreatitis. *World J Emerg Surg.* 2019;14:27.

6. Balthazar EJ. Acute pancreatitis: assessment of severity with clinical and CT evaluation. *Radiology.* 2002;223:603–613.

7. Tenner S, Baillie J, DeWitt J, Vege SS. American College of Gastroenterology guideline: management of acute pancreatitis. *Am J Gastroenterol.* 2013;108(9):1400–1415. 1416.

8. *Imipenem/Cilastatin.* Reference.medscape.com.

9. *Piperacillin/Tazobactam.* Reference.medscape.com.

10. *Ticarcillin/Clavulanate.* Reference.medscape.com.

11. *Ceftazidime.* Reference.medscape.com.

12. *Cefuroxime.* Reference.medscape.com.

13. Twilla JD, Mancell J. Hypertriglyceridemia-induced acute pancreatitis treated with insulin and heparin. *Am J Health Syst Pharm.* 2012;69(3):213–216.

Acute Ischemic Colitis

Presentation

Ischemic colitis is the most common form of gastrointestinal ischemia.[1] This condition is caused by decreased blood flow to the colon. Most cases of ischemia are transient and usually do not lead to full-thickness necrosis. Most ischemic colitis cases can be managed with conservative treatment. The left colon is most commonly affected; however, the right ischemic colon is associated with a higher mortality rate.[1]

Patients older than 65 and with hypercoagulable conditions and cardiac arrhythmias are at higher risk. Causes of ischemic colitis include emboli, thrombosis, small vessel disease, vasculitis, and shock.[1]

Symptoms include acute onset abdominal pain/cramping, urgent desire to defecate, bright red or maroon blood per rectum within first 24 h. If colonic necrosis becomes transmural, patients will develop peritoneal signs on abdominal examination, such as guarding and rebound tenderness.

Causes for Rapid Response Activation

Tachycardia, tachypnea, hypotension, and altered mental status in patients who develop bowel necrosis.

Actions

INITIAL MEASURES

1. Maintain continuous pulse oximetry
2. Administer supplemental oxygen to maintain SpO_2 of 96%–99%
3. Maintain continuous cardiac monitoring and blood pressure measurements

DIAGNOSTIC WORK-UP

1. Labs: CBC with differential (anemia, leukocytosis, bandemia), complete metabolic panel (electrolyte abnormalities, elevated creatinine, metabolic acidosis, low albumin), PT, aPTT, INR, D-dimer (elevated), lactic acid (elevated), and thrombophilia panel if hypercoagulable state is suspected.
2. CT scan of abdomen and pelvis with IV and oral contrast is imaging of choice and is useful to assess the distribution of colitis; it will show bowel wall thickening, edema, and thumbprinting; colonic pneumatosis or portomesenteric venous gas predicts the presence of transmural colonic infarction.[2]
3. Early colonoscopy within 48 h of presentation should be performed in suspected ischemic colitis cases to confirm the diagnosis:
   - The colon should be insufflated minimally.
   - Colonoscopy should be stopped at the distal-most extent of the disease.

- Biopsies of the colonic mucosa should be obtained except in cases of gangrene.
- Colonoscopy should not be done in patients with acute peritonitis or irreversible isch-emic damage such as gangrene and pneumatosis.[3]

TREATMENT

1. Start aggressive IV fluid resuscitation with isotonic sodium chloride and blood products if indicated.
2. Vasopressors should be avoided as they can worsen ischemia; however, for patients with severe hypotension refractory to aggressive IV fluid resuscitation, may consider norepi-nephrine with caution:
   - Norepinephrine 0.03–3 μk/kg/min IV.[4]
3. Correct electrolytes.
4. Administer broad spectrum antibiotics that cover both aerobic and anaerobic coliform bacteria.
5. Start intubation and mechanical ventilation for unstable patients.
6. In patients who develop pancolonic ischemic colitis, worsening peritonitis, perforated viscous, uncontrolled bleeding, hemodynamic instability, or failure to improve, surgical intervention is required and bowel resection is performed; definitive surgical interventions include:
   - End colostomy and rectal stump (Hartmann procedure) is used for left-sided ischemic colitis.
   - Resection with primary anastomosis is preferred for right colon ischemia with no evi-dence of perforation.[5]

References

1. Washington C, Carmichael JC. Management of ischemic colitis. *Clin Colon Rectal Surg.* 2012;25(4):228–235.
2. Milone M, Di Minno MN, Musella M, et al. Computed tomography findings of pneumatosis and porto-mesenteric venous gas in acute bowel ischemia. *World J Gastroenterol.* 2013;19(39):6579–6584.
3. Brandt LJ, Feuerstadt P, Longstreth GF, Boley SJ. ACG clinical guideline: epidemiology, risk factors, pat-terns of presentation, diagnosis, and management of colon ischemia. *Am J Gastroenterol.* 2015;110(1):18–44.
4. Rollstin A, Chiu WC, Marshall JP. Vasopressor and inotropes. *Critical Care Emergency Medicine.* 2nd ed. McGrawHill Education; vol. 19; 2017:193–200.
5. Gandhi SK, Hanson MM, Vernava AM, et al. Ischemic colitis. *Dis Colon Rectum.* 1996;39(6):1171–1174.

Acute Mesenteric Ischemia

Presentation

Mesenteric ischemia is uncommon with prevalence of 0.09%–0.2% of all hospital admissions in the United States.[1] Mesenteric ischemia is a sudden onset of small intestinal hypoperfusion that occurs due to obstruction of the arteries or veins of the small intestine. Obstruction can occur due to arterial emboli, arterial thrombi, venous thrombi, or vasospasm of the superior mesenteric artery (SMA).

Elderly patients are at risk for acute mesenteric ischemia. Arterial embolisms can be caused by emboli lodged in the superior mesenteric artery. Patients with atrial fibrillation, recent angiography, vasculitis, cardiomyopathy, and valvular heart disease are at high risk. Risk factors for mesenteric arterial thrombosis include atherosclerosis, peripheral arterial disease, prolonged hypotension, estrogen therapy, or hypercoagulability. Conditions that cause resistance for mesenteric venous blood outflow, such as inflammatory bowel disease, increase risk for mesenteric venous thrombosis. Nonocclusive mesenteric ischemia may occur due to the SMA spasm in the setting of shock, vasoconstrictive medications, or cocaine abuse.

Symptoms of mesenteric arterial embolism include anorexia, nausea, vomiting, diarrhea, blood in stool, abdominal distention, and sudden onset of severe abdominal pain. Pain can be out of proportion to abdominal examination.

Symptoms of mesenteric arterial thrombosis include abdominal angina described as severe abdominal pain, usually 15–20 min after eating and lasting for 1–3 h. Pain is progressively worse.

Symptoms of mesenteric venous thrombosis include abdominal pain with more insidious onset. These patients are usually younger and have inherited hypercoagulable conditions, take oral contraceptive pills, or have liver disease or malignancy.

Morbidity and mortality associated with acute mesenteric ischemia is high if untreated and can cause intestinal necrosis, perforation, and death.

Causes for Rapid Response Activation

Tachycardia, tachypnea, hypotension, and altered mental status in patients who develop bowel necrosis.

Actions

INITIAL MEASURES

1. Maintain continuous pulse oximetry
2. Administer supplemental oxygen to maintain SpO_2 of 96%–99%
3. Maintain continuous cardiac monitoring and blood pressure measurements
4. Consult with general or vascular surgeon early in the course of rapid response

DIAGNOSTIC WORK-UP

1. Labs: CBC with differential (leukocytosis, bandemia), complete metabolic panel (electrolyte abnormalities, elevated creatinine, metabolic acidosis), coagulation studies (PT, aPTT, INR), D-dimer (elevated), lactic acid (elevated), amylase (elevated), and thrombophilia panel if hypercoagulable state is suspected.
2. CT angiography is initial diagnostic imaging.

TREATMENT

1. Order bowel rest.
2. Consider NG tube placement for patients with ileus.
3. Start aggressive IV fluid resuscitation with isotonic sodium chloride and blood products if indicated.
4. Vasopressors should be avoided as they can worsen ischemia; however, for patients with severe hypotension refractory to aggressive IV fluid resuscitation, may consider norepinephrine with caution:
   - Norepinephrine 0.03–3 µg/kg/min IV[2]
5. Correct electrolytes.
6. Administer broad spectrum antibiotics in patients with bowel ischemia.
7. Start intubation and mechanical ventilation for unstable patients.
8. Treatment should be prompt; consult general or vascular surgeon promptly to consider:
   - Surgical laparotomy with embolectomy for mesenteric arterial embolism
   - Exploratory laparotomy for surgical revascularization such as aorta to superior mesenteric arterial bypass grafting or reimplantation of the superior mesenteric artery into the aorta for mesenteric arterial thrombosis[3]
9. Administer systemic anticoagulation therapy, for example, heparin drip either alone or in combination with exploratory laparotomy, for mesenteric venous thrombosis; start heparin at a bolus of 80 U/kg, not to exceed 5000 U, followed by 18 U/kg/h until therapeutic INR of 2–3 is achieved with oral warfarin; monitor the activated partial thromboplastin time (aPTT).[4]
10. Most patients will require a second-look laparotomy 24–48 h after mesenteric revascularization to reassess the viability of the small intestine.
11. Continue long-term systemic anticoagulation after discharge from hospital.
12. Ensure surveillance of the mesenteric artery stent with duplex ultrasound or CT angiography.

References

1. Chaudhry R, Zaki J, Wegner R, et al. Gastrointestinal complications after cardiac surgery: a nationwide population-based analysis of morbidity and mortality predictors. *J Cardiothorac Vasc Anesth.* 2017;31(4):1268–1274.
2. Rollstin A, Chiu WC, Marshall JP. Vasopressor and inotropes. *Critical Care Emergency Medicine.* 2nd ed. McGrawHill Education; vol. 19; 2017:193–200.
3. Tambyraja AL. Management of acute mesenteric ischaemia: recommended strategy is misleading. *BMJ.* 2003;327(7411):396.
4. Dang CV. *Acute Mesenteric Ischemia, Treatment and Management.* Emedicine.medscape.com. Updated: March 26, 2020; 2020.

CHAPTER 5

Endocrine Emergencies

Severe Diabetic Ketoacidosis

Presentation

Diabetic ketoacidosis (DKA) is a serious acute metabolic complication of diabetes and is characterized by the triad of severe hyperglycemia, metabolic acidosis, and elevated total body ketone production. DKA can occur both in DM type I (2/3 of cases) and in DM type II (1/3 of cases). The diagnosis of severe diabetic ketoacidosis is confirmed by elevated serum ketones, serum bicarb < 10 mEq/L, elevated anion gap > 12 mEq/L, and arterial pH < 7.[1] DKA can be precipitated by infection (most common cause), noncompliance with treatment, surgery, or trauma.

Symptoms include generalized weakness, polydipsia, polyphagia, polyuria, weight loss, nausea, vomiting, and abdominal pain. Signs include dry mucous membranes, flattened neck veins, tachypnea, tachycardia, and hypotension.

Causes for Rapid Response Activation

Tachycardia, hypotension, decreased consciousness, stupor, coma.

Actions

INITIAL MEASURES

1. Maintain continuous pulse oximetry.
2. Administer supplemental oxygen to maintain $SpO_2 > 95\%$.
3. Maintain continuous cardiac monitoring/blood pressure measurements.

DIAGNOSTIC WORK-UP

1. ABG (to assess severity of metabolic acidosis)
2. Labs: CBC with differential (bandemia is more predictable of infection than leukocytosis), procalcitonin (elevated in bacterial and fungal infection), CMP, serum phosphate, magnesium, serum ketone, A1C, and UA (glucosuria, ketones, UTI)
3. Chest X-ray to rule out infiltrate consistent with pneumonia
4. EKG to assess potassium effect, arrhythmias, MI

TREATMENT

1. Start IVF resuscitation, such as 0.9% saline 1000–1500 mL IV within the first hour, followed by maintenance fluids, such as 0.9% saline if corrected serum sodium is low or 0.45% saline usually at 250–500 mL/h (patients are generally depleted at 3–6 L in DKA);

monitor heart rate, blood pressure, urine output, and respiratory status; use caution with heart failure and renal failure patients—avoid fluid overload.[2]

2. Add 5% dextrose IV when blood sugar is ≤ 200 mg/dL to allow continued insulin administration until anion gap is closed and ketonemia is controlled.

3. Maintain continuous IV regular insulin infusion:
   ▪ Administer IV bolus of regular insulin at 0.1 units/kg, followed by a continuous infusion of regular insulin at a dose of 0.1 units/kg/h; or
   ▪ IV regular insulin at 0.14 units/kg/h, for example, 10 units/h for a 70-kg patient.
   ▪ Goal is to decrease plasma glucose by 50–75 mg/dL in 1 h period.
   ▪ Decrease insulin by 50% if blood glucose decreases by > 75 mg/dL in 1 h period.
   ▪ Increase insulin by 50% if blood glucose decreases by < 50 mg/dL in 1 h period.
   ▪ If blood glucose decreases by 50–75 mg/dL in 1 h period, keep insulin at the same rate.
   ▪ When blood glucose decreases to 200 mg/dL, decrease insulin infusion rate to 0.02–0.05 units/kg/h and add 5% dextrose IV.
   ▪ Continue insulin infusion to maintain plasma glucose between 150 and 200 mg/dL in DKA until resolution of DKA.[2]

4. In patients with a pH < 6.9, start 100 mEq of sodium bicarbonate in 400 mL of sterile water with 20 mEq of potassium chloride at a rate of 200 mL/h for 2 h; should be repeated every 2 h until the patient's pH is 6.9 or greater.[2]

5. Start potassium supplementation:
   ▪ If serum K is > 5.2 mEq/L—leave potassium out of IVF, but check serum potassium level q 2 h.
   ▪ If serum K is 3.3–5.2 mEq/L—add 20–30 mEq KCl/L of IVF for goal serum potassium of 4–5 mEq/L.
   ▪ If serum K is < 3.3—hold insulin to prevent cardiac arrhythmias; administer 20–30 mEq KCl/L of IVF, and start insulin drip when K > 3.3 mEq/L.[2]

6. In patients with serum phosphate < 1 mg/dL, in patients with anemia, respiratory depression, or cardiac dysfunction, add 20–30 mEq of potassium phosphate/L of IVF.[2]

7. In patients with magnesium < 1.2 mg/dL, treat with magnesium sulfate 2 g IV.

8. DKA is resolved when:
   ▪ Anion gap ≤ 12 mEq/L
   ▪ Plasma glucose level < 200 mg/dL
   ▪ Venous pH > 7.3
   ▪ Bicarbonate level ≥ 15 mEq/L[2]

9. Once these levels are achieved and oral fluids are tolerated, convert insulin drip to a long-acting subcutaneous form of insulin in combination with a correctional short-acting insulin sliding scale.

10. Start home insulin dose; those new to insulin should receive 0.5–0.8 U/kg/day in divided doses.

11. IV insulin drip should remain in place for 2 h after subcutaneous insulin is initiated.

12. Determine the precipitating cause of DKA, such as infection, inadequate insulin treatment, noncompliance with insulin treatment, pancreatitis, acute coronary syndrome, stroke, drugs, or pregnancy.[3]

References

1. Kitabchi AE, Umpierrez GE, Murphy MB, et al. Hyperglycemic crises in diabetes. *Diabetes Care.* 2004;27(1):S94–102.
2. Kitabchi AE, Umpierrez GE, Miles JM, Fisher JN. Hyperglycemic crisis in adult patients with diabetes. *Diabetes Care.* 2009;32(7):1335–1343.
3. Dyanne P, Westerberg DO. Diabetic ketoacidosis: evaluation and treatment. *Am Fam Physician.* 2013;87(5):337–346.

Hyperosmolar Hyperglycemic State

Presentation

Occurs in DM type II. Usually precipitated by lack of access to water in chronically ill elderly patients with diminished thirst perception. Symptoms include profound dehydration, headache, weakness, polyuria, polydipsia, nausea, vomiting, abdominal pain, lethargy, stupor, and coma.

Blood glucose is more elevated compared to DKA, such as $> 600 \, mg/dL$; therefore, serum osmolality is $> 330–380 \, mOsm/kg$. Unlike DKA, in HHS, $pH > 7.3$, serum bicarb $> 20 \, mEq/L$, anion gap is normal < 12, serum potassium is normal, and there is more severe elevation in serum creatinine.[1]

Causes for Rapid Response Activation

Tachycardia, hypotension, stupor, coma, seizures.

Actions

INITIAL MEASURES

1. Maintain continuous pulse oximetry.
2. Administer supplemental oxygen to maintain $SpO_2 > 95\%$.
3. Maintain continuous cardiac monitoring/blood pressure measurements.

DIAGNOSTIC WORK-UP

1. Labs: ABG, serum osmolality, CBC with differential (bandemia is more predictable of infection than leukocytosis), procalcitonin (elevated in bacterial/fungal infection), CMP, serum phosphate, magnesium, serum ketone, A1C, and UA (glucosuria, ketones, UTI)
2. Chest X-ray (infiltrate consistent with pneumonia)
3. EKG (to assess ischemia or arrhythmia)

TREATMENT

1. Start IVF resuscitation such as 0.9% saline 1000–1500 mL IV within the first hour, followed by maintenance fluids such as 0.9% saline if corrected serum sodium is low or 0.45% saline, usually at 250–500 mL/h (patients are generally depleted at 8–12 L in HHS); monitor heart rate, blood pressure, urine output, and respiratory status; use caution with heart failure and renal failure patients—avoid fluid overload.[2]
2. Add 5% dextrose IV when blood sugar is $< 300 \, mg/dL$.[2]
3. Maintain continuous IV of regular insulin infusion:
   - Administer IV bolus of regular insulin at 0.1 units/kg, followed by a continuous infusion of regular insulin at a dose of 0.1 units/kg/h; or
   - IV regular insulin at 0.14 units/kg/h, for example, 10 units/h for a 70-kg patient.
   - Goal is to decrease plasma glucose by 50–75 mg/dL in 1 h period.

- Decrease insulin by 50% if blood glucose decreases by > 75 mg/dL in 1 h period.
- Increase insulin by 50% if blood glucose decreases by < 50 mg/dL in 1 h period.
- If blood glucose decreases by 50–75 mg/dL in 1 h period, keep insulin at the same rate.
- When blood glucose decreases to 300 mg/dL, decrease insulin infusion rate to 0.02–0.05 units/kg/h and add 5% dextrose IV.[2]

4. Continue insulin infusion to maintain plasma glucose between 200 and 300 mg/dL in HHS until resolution of HHS.[2]
5. HHS is resolved when:
   - Mental status is normalized
   - Serum osmolality is < 320
   - Patient is able to tolerate PO intake[2]
6. When the preceding goals are achieved, convert insulin drip to a long-acting subcutaneous form of insulin in combination with a correctional short-acting insulin sliding scale.
7. Start home insulin dose; those new to insulin should receive 0.5–0.8 U/kg/day in divided doses.
8. IV insulin drip should remain in place for 2 h after subcutaneous insulin is initiated.
9. In patients with serum phosphate < 1 mg/dL or in patients with anemia, respiratory depression, or cardiac dysfunction, add 20–30 mEq of potassium phosphate/L of IVF.[2]
10. In patients with magnesium < 1.2 mg/dL, treat with magnesium sulfate 2 g IV.
11. Determine the precipitating cause of HHS, such as infection, inadequate insulin treatment, noncompliance with insulin treatment, pancreatitis, acute coronary syndrome, stroke, drugs (atypical antipsychotics, corticosteroids), or alcohol abuse.

References

1. Stoner GD. Hyperosmolar hyperglycemic state. *Am Fam Physician.* 2017;96(11):729–736.
2. Kitabchi AE, Umpierrez GE, Miles JM, Fisher JN. Hyperglycemic crisis in adult patients with diabetes. *Diabetes Care.* 2009;32(7):1335–1343.

Hyperthyroidism/Thyroid Storm

Presentation

Thyroid storm is an acute hyperthyroid state due to excessive release of thyroid hormones resulting in end-organ dysfunction. Thyroid storm can be precipitated by sepsis, thyroidectomy, nonthyroidal surgery, anesthesia induction, abrupt cessation of antithyroid drug therapy, anticholinergic drugs, adrenergic drugs, and chemotherapy. Diagnosis of thyroid storm is made clinically.[1,2]

Symptoms include high fever, diaphoresis, altered mental status, dyspnea, nausea, vomiting, diarrhea, and abdominal pain. On examination, patients can have lid lag, hyperreflexia, tachycardia, and cardiac arrhythmias such as atrial fibrillation, hypertension, and tachypnea. Hypertension and tachycardia may be followed by high output acute decompensated heart failure.[3]

Causes for Rapid Response Activation

Severe dyspnea, cardiac arrhythmias, progressively worsening neurological status, such as agitation, delirium, seizure, coma, or psychosis.

Actions

INITIAL MEASURES

1. Maintain continuous pulse oximetry.
2. Administer supplemental oxygen to maintain $SpO_2 > 95\%$.
3. Maintain continuous cardiac monitoring/blood pressure measurements.
4. Transfer to ICU.
5. Assess patient with a Burch-Wartofsky Point Scale (BWPS), which includes temperature, tachycardia, atrial fibrillation, and congestive heart failure:
   - ≥ 45 points is consistent with thyroid storm.
   - 25–44 points is consistent with impending thyroid storm.
   - < 25 points make thyroid storm unlikely.[2]
6. Consult endocrinologist early in the course of rapid response.

DIAGNOSTIC WORK-UP

1. Labs: Thyroid function tests (will show undetectable TSH and elevated free T4 and free T3), CBC (leukocytosis), BMP (hypercalcemia), magnesium, baseline liver panel, and ABG.
2. Chest X-ray may demonstrate signs of congestive heart failure and pulmonary edema.
3. EKG: The most common arrhythmia associated with thyroid storm is atrial fibrillation; other cardiac arrhythmias include atrial flutter and ventricular arrhythmias.
4. Head CT scan may be considered to exclude other causes of altered mental status.

TREATMENT

1. Use cooling measures, for example, cooling blankets/antipyretics such as rectal acetaminophen.
2. Start IV fluid replacement in hypovolemic patients.
3. Correct electrolyte abnormalities.
4. May treat agitation with haloperidol.
5. Administer thionamides:
   - Propylthiouracil 600–1000 mg loading dose, followed by 200–250 mg every 4–6 h orally, via nasogastric tube, or rectally to block peripheral conversion of T4 to T3; monitor for liver toxicity; switch to methimazole at the time of discharge, unless methimazole is contraindicated, in which case, consider radioactive iodine or surgery.[2]
   - Methimazole 20 mg every 6 h orally, through nasogastric tube, or rectally.[2]
6. In patients with Graves' disease who have adverse reaction to thionamides, consider iodine (saturated solution of potassium iodide) five drops (0.25 mL or 250 mg) orally or via nasogastric tube every 6 h; treat for about a week in preparation for thyroidectomy.
7. Administer beta-blockers to reduce tachycardia and hypertension:[2]
   - Propranolol 1–2 mg/min IV q 15 min up to max 10 mg[1]
   - Esmolol as a loading dose of 250–500 µg/kg, followed by an infusion of 50–100 µg/kg/min[1]
8. Administer hydrocortisone 100 mg IV every 6–8 h to reduce thyroid hormone release.[2, 3]
9. In refractory cases, consult nephrology for plasmapheresis or peritoneal hemodialysis to remove circulating thyroid hormone.

References

1. Carroll R, Matfin G. Endocrine and metabolic emergencies: thyroid storm. *Ther Adv Endocrinol Metab.* 2010;1(3):139–145.
2. Ross DS, Burch HB, Cooper DS, et al. 2016 American Thyroid Association Guidelines for diagnosis and management of hyperthyroidism and other causes of thyrotoxicosis. *Thyroid.* 2016;26(10):1343–1421.
3. Misra M, Hoffman RP, et al. *Thyroid Storm Treatment and Management.* Emedicine.medscape.com. Updated: March 16, 2020.

Hypothryroidism/Myxedema Coma

Presentation

Myxedema coma is a rare life-threatening condition in patients with long-standing untreated hypothyroidism. Usually occurs in patients 60 years or older. Myxedema coma mostly occurs during winter, as cold exposure is one of the important precipitating factors.

Precipitating factors also include infection, drugs (sedatives, analgesics, diuretics), stroke, myocardial infarction, congestive heart failure, gastrointestinal bleeding, and trauma.

Symptoms include periorbital edema, ptosis, macroglossia, altered mental status, skin and soft tissue swelling. On physical examination, patients may have hypothermia, bradycardia, or hypotension.[1]

Causes for Rapid Response Activation

Bradycardia, hypotension, deterioration of mental status such as obtundation, stupor, coma.

Actions

INITIAL MEASURES

1. Maintain continuous pulse oximetry.
2. Administer supplemental oxygen to maintain $SpO_2 > 95\%$.
3. Maintain continuous cardiac monitoring/blood pressure measurements.

DIAGNOSTIC WORK-UP

1. Labs: CBC (anemia, leukopenia), CMP (hyponatremia, elevated creatinine, hypercapnia, hypoglycemia, elevated transaminases), procalcitonin (elevated in bacterial/fungal infections), serum osmolality (low), CPK (elevated); thyroid function tests will usually show elevated TSH and undetectable free T4 and free T3.
2. EKG will assess the effects of electrolyte abnormalities.

TREATMENT

1. Use regular blankets to warm patients with hypothermia; avoid warming blankets as they can cause peripheral vascular dilation and hemodynamic instability; monitor temperature with a rectal probe.[1]
2. Start cautious IVF resuscitation with 0.9% saline; avoid vasopressors if possible as they can cause arrhythmias and ischemia in the setting of IV thyroxine[1]; if vasopressors are necessary, consider dopamine 5–15 µg/kg/min IV.[2]
3. Correct electrolyte abnormalities.
4. Administer dexamethasone 2–4 mg IV every 12 h for possible concomitant adrenal insufficiency (as administration of thyroid hormones will increase metabolism and hepatic clearance of cortisol); dexamethasone does not affect the serum cortisol concentration and can be used without affecting the results of the cosyntropin test.[3]

5. Check random cortisol level:
   - Cortisol level is > 23 µg/dL: discontinue dexamethasone.
   - Cortisol level is < 3 µg/dL: either continue dexamethasone or switch to hydrocortisone 100 mg IV every 8 h.
   - Cortisol level is 3–23 µg/dL: proceed with cosyntropin test.[4]
6. For cosyntropin test, administer cosyntropin (synthetic ACTH) 250 µg IV; then measure cortisol level at 30 and 60 min postinfusion; high cortisol level of > 20 µg/dL can exclude the diagnosis of adrenal insufficiency.[5]
7. Administer high-dose intravenous thyroxine as a bolus of 200–400 µg, followed by 1.6 µg/kg daily[5]; a smaller dose may be given to smaller patients, older patients, and patients with history of cardiac arrhythmias or coronary artery disease.
8. Measure thyroid hormones every 1–2 days.[6]
9. Failure of TSH to trend down is an indication to either increase the dose of levothyroxine or add liothyronine at a loading dose of 5–20 µg, followed by a maintenance dose of 2.5–10 µg every 8 h, with lower doses for smaller patients, older patients, and patients with a history of cardiac arrhythmias or coronary artery disease; continue liothyronine until therapeutic endpoints have been achieved, such as improved mental status.[6]
10. IV levothyroxine may lead to improvement within 1 week in the following aspects:
    - Mental status
    - Cardiac function
    - Pulmonary function
    - Renal function
    - Metabolic parameters[6]
11. When patient is fully awake and is able to have oral intake, switch to oral levothyroxine.
12. Determine and treat the precipitating causes of myxedema coma, such as infection, acute coronary syndrome, and trauma.

References

1. Wal CR. Myxedema coma: diagnosis and treatment. *Am Fam Physician.* 2000;62(11):2485–2490.
2. *Dopamine.* Reference.medscape.com.
3. Eledrisi MS, et al. *Myxedema Coma or Crisis*; 2020. Emedicine.medscape.com.
4. Griffing GT. *Serum Cortisol*; 2019. Emedicine.medscape.com.
5. Hamilton DD, Cotton BA. Cosyntropin as a diagnostic agent in the screening of patients for adrenocortical insufficiency. *Clin Pharmacol.* 2010;2:77–82.
6. Jonclaas J, Bianco AC, Bauer AJ, et al. Guidelines for the treatment of hypothyroidism. American Thyroid Association Task Force on Thyroid Hormone Replacement. *Thyroid.* 2014;24(12):1670–1751.

Acute Adrenal (Addisonian) Crisis

Presentation

Acute adrenal crisis is a life-threatening condition caused by severe cortisol insufficiency. It can occur as a result of previously undiagnosed or untreated adrenal failure. Adrenal crisis can also occur in patients with known adrenal insufficiency when there is a cessation in the amount of cortisol needed to meet the increased need for cortisol, for example, due to illness, trauma, surgery, or childbirth.[1]

Symptoms include severe weakness, anorexia, nausea, vomiting, diarrhea, abdominal pain, muscle/joint pain, confusion, lethargy, and delirium. On physical examination, patients may have skin and mucosal hyperpigmentation, tachycardia, or hypotension.[1]

Causes for Rapid Response Activation

Cardiac arrhythmias, hypovolemic shock, tachypnea, decreased consciousness, seizure.

Actions

INITIAL MEASURES

1. Maintain continuous pulse oximetry.
2. Administer supplemental oxygen to maintain $SpO_2 > 95\%$.
3. Maintain continuous cardiac monitoring/blood pressure measurements.
4. Transfer hemodynamically unstable patients to ICU.
5. Start immediate therapeutic intervention prior to confirmation of the diagnosis with baseline cortisol level.

DIAGNOSTIC WORK-UP

1. Labs: CBC (leukocytosis, eosinophilia), BMP (hyponatremia, hyperkalemia, hypoglycemia, hypercalcemia, elevated creatinine), venous blood gas (metabolic acidosis); in patients with no known diagnosis of adrenal insufficiency, order serum cortisol, ACTH, aldosterone, renin, and cosyntropin stimulation test.
2. Cosyntropin test: administer cosyntropin (synthetic ACTH) 250 µg IV; then measure cortisol level at 30 and 60 min postinfusion; high cortisol level of > 20 µg/dL can exclude the diagnosis of adrenal insufficiency.[2]
3. Chest X-ray may demonstrate lymphoma, metastases, sarcoid, histoplasmosis, or tuberculosis.
4. CT scan of abdomen may show adrenal hemorrhage, metastases, or atrophy.

TREATMENT

1. Start IVF resuscitation with 1000 mL of normal saline IV bolus within first hour,[1] followed by maintenance fluids guided by hemodynamic monitoring, for example, urine output (normal urine output is 0.5–1.5 mL/kg/h); avoid rapid correction of hyponatremia (more than 6–8 mEq in the first 24 h) to avoid osmotic demyelination syndrome.[3]
2. Monitor blood glucose frequently and start 5%–10% dextrose IV in hypoglycemia.[1]
3. Start vasopressor in patients with hypotension refractory to IVF resuscitation:
   - Norepinephrine 0.03–3.0 µg/kg/min IV infusion[4]
   - Dopamine 5–20 µg/kg/min IV infusion[4]
4. Administer stress dose steroids:
   - Hydrocortisone 50 mg IV every 6 h for 2–3 days[1]
   - Fludrocortisone acetate 0.05–0.2 mg IV daily with subsequent tapering of hydrocortisone dose[1]
5. Replace electrolytes.
6. Determine the precipitating cause of acute adrenal crisis, such as infection, acute coronary syndrome, or trauma.
7. Consult endocrinologist early in the course of rapid response.

References

1. Puar T, Stikkelbroek N, Smans L, et al. Adrenal crisis: still a deadly event in the 21st century. *Am J Med.* 2016;129(3). 339.E1–339.E9.
2. Hamilton DD, Cotton BA. Cosyntropin as a diagnostic agent in the screening of patients for adrenocortical insufficiency. *Clin Pharmacol.* 2010;2:77–82.
3. Verbalis JG, Goldsmith SR, Greenberg A, et al. Diagnosis, evaluation, and treatment of hyponatremia: expert panel recommendations. *Am J Med.* 2013;126(10):1. S1–S42.
4. Rollstin A, Chiu WC, Marshall JP. Vasopressors and inotropes. *Critical Care Emergency Medicine*; 2nd ed. McGrawHill Education; 2017:193–200. Chapter 19.

Hypercalcemic Crisis

Presentation

Elevation of serum calcium > 14 mg/dL.[1] The most common cause of hypercalcemia is primary hyperparathyroidism due to benign parathyroid adenoma, which leads to excessive secretion of PTH (parathyroid hormone). Parathyroid carcinoma can also increase serum PTH level. PTH leads to hypercalcemia via osteoclastic bone resorption. The next most common etiology for hypercalcemia is malignancy. Multiple bone metastases cause hypercalcemia by osteolysis, or hypercalcemia can be caused by parathyroid hormone–related protein (PTHrP) secretion.[1]

Symptoms include fatigue, headache, nausea, vomiting, abdominal/flank pain, constipation, and polyuria. Severe symptoms include obtundation, stupor, and coma. Hypercalcemic crisis can lead to severe necrotizing pancreatitis. Hypercalcemia can shorten QT interval and cause cardiac arrhythmias such as complete heart block and cardiac arrest. Other causes of hypercalcemia include immobilization, medications like thiazides or lithium, granulomatous diseases like sarcoidosis or tuberculosis, hyperthyroidism, and adrenal insufficiency.[1]

Causes for Rapid Response Activation

Progressively worsening mental status or cardiac arrhythmias such as complete heart block.

Actions

INITIAL MEASURES

1. Maintain continuous pulse oximetry.
2. Administer supplemental oxygen to maintain SpO_2 > 95%.
3. Maintain continuous cardiac monitoring/blood pressure measurements.

DIAGNOSTIC WORK-UP

1. Labs: BMP, magnesium, phosphorus, albumin to calculate corrected total calcium, ionized calcium, digoxin level if patient is taking digoxin, and serum PTH and PTHrP.
2. Order EKG to check QT interval shortening and prolongation of PR interval; at very high levels—lengthening of QRS interval, flattening or inversion of T waves, and a variable degree of heart block; digoxin may worsen these findings.
3. Chest X-ray may show malignancy or sarcoidosis.
4. Start intravascular volume expansion with isotonic crystalloid, for example, 0.9% normal saline, as these patients are hypovolemic due to hypercalcemia–induced polyuria.
5. Loop diuretic, for example, furosemide, may be used with hydration to increase calcium excretion; however, avoid in severely dehydrated patients.
6. In patients with advanced renal failure to the point that diuresis is impossible, hydration will be ineffective; therefore, they will need hemodialysis; consult nephrologist in this case.
7. Administer bisphosphonate therapy with close monitoring of renal function due to risk of renal injury; may take 48–72 h before reaching full therapeutic effect[2]:

- Pamidronate 90 mg IV over 2–24 h; longer infusions in patients with preexisting CKD to prevent renal toxicity;[3] may repeat the dose in 7 days as needed.
- Zoledronate 4 mg IV over 15 min, may repeat the dose in 7 days as needed.[4]

8. Surgery is advisable for primary hyperparathyroidism.
9. Consult oncologist to address malignancies.

References

1. Ahmad S, Kuraganti G, Steenkamp D. Hypercalcemic crisis: a clinical review. *Am J Med*. 2015;128(3):239–245.
2. Cho KC. Electrolyte and acid-base disorders. In: *Current Medical Diagnosis and Treatment*; 2nd ed. McGrawHill Education; 2013. Chapter 21.
3. *Pamidronate*. Reference.medscape.com.
4. *Zoledronic Acid*. Reference.medscape.com.

Hypocalcemic Crisis

Presentation

Hypocalcemia is usually due to an inadequate parathyroid hormone or vitamin D level or resistance to them. Severe hypocalcemia (<0.9 mmol/L of ionized calcium)[1] is associated with critical illness. Hypocalcemia is very common in critically ill patients (55%), and severe hypocalcemia may occur in up to 6% of ICU patients.[1] Patients with severe hypocalcemia who fail to normalize their ionized calcium have higher mortality risk.

Other causes of hypocalcemia include postparathyroidectomy hungry bone disease, hypoparathyroidism due to autoimmune disease, history of radiation of parathyroid glands, end-stage renal disease or end-stage liver disease causing a vitamin D deficiency, or drugs such as diuretics, antiepileptics, and cisplatin.

Symptoms include paresthesia, circumoral numbness, muscle spasms/cramps (tetany), seizure, refractory hypotension, and arrhythmias.

Causes for Rapid Response Activation

Seizure, laryngeal tetany causing difficulty breathing, hypotension, cardiac arrhythmias.

Actions

INITIAL MEASURES

1. Maintain continuous pulse oximetry.
2. Administer supplemental oxygen to maintain $SpO_2 > 95\%$.
3. Maintain continuous cardiac monitoring/blood pressure measurements.

DIAGNOSTIC WORK-UP

1. Labs: BMP, magnesium, phosphorus (elevated), albumin to calculate corrected total calcium, ionized calcium, PTH (low), 1,25-dihydroxyvitamin D_3 level (low), digoxin level in patients taking digoxin as calcium potentiates digitalis toxicity.
2. EKG: prolonged QT-interval.

TREATMENT

1. Start IVF replacement therapy.
2. Administer calcium gluconate:
   - Without seizure or tetany: 0.5 mg/kg/h IV[2]
   - With tetany or seizure: 1–3 g IV, followed by infusion drip at 0.5 mg/kg/h
   - May titrate up to 2 mg/kg/h to maintain serum calcium level at 8–9 mg/dL; avoid rapid correction of calcium as this can contribute into cardiac arrhythmias such as bradycardia or hypotension[2]
3. Central venous catheter is preferred to avoid extravasation and irritation of tissue.

4. Check serum calcium level every 4–6 h; may check ionized calcium in patients with hypoalbuminemia.
5. Continuous cardiac monitoring during IV calcium supplementation is especially necessary in patients taking digoxin therapy.
6. Start oral calcium and vitamin D supplementation early.

References

1. Steele T, Kolamunnage-Dona R, Downey C. Assessment and clinical course of hypocalcemia in critical illness. *Crit Care*. 2013;17(3):R106.
2. Suneja M. *Hypocalcemia Treatment and Management*. Emedicine.medcape.com. Updated: August 08, 2019.

Acute Severe Hypernatremia

Presentation

Acute hypernatremia is associated with sodium > 158 mmol/L within < 48 h and is symptomatic.[1] Hypernatremia commonly occurs in critically ill patients in ICU. Elderly patients, especially with altered mental status or infection, are at high risk. Hypernatremia can cause a shift of free water from intracellular to extracellular space, which can lead to cerebral cell shrinkage followed by vascular rupture causing intracerebral bleeding. Severe hypernatremia can also cause rhabdomyolysis and subsequent acute kidney failure. Loss of volume can cause circulatory problems such as tachycardia and hypotension.

Hypernatremia is due to sodium gain or water loss. Causes of sodium gain may be due to the administration of hypertonic solutions such as sodium bicarbonate, use of large volumes of saline during resuscitation of patients with multiorgan failure, sodium-rich antibiotics such as ciprofloxacin, ticarcillin, fluconazole, and voriconazole, among others.

There are renal and extrarenal causes of water loss. Renal water loss is due to osmotic diuresis secondary to hyperglycemia/glucosuria (diabetes mellitus), urea (high protein tube feedings), and mannitol. Loop diuretics can also cause renal water loss. Central (head injury/surgery) and nephrogenic diabetes insipidus (drugs such as contrast media, lithium, rifampin, foscarnet, amphotericin B; ethanol; hypercalcemia) are other causes of renal water loss. Extrarenal water loss can be due to fever, vomiting, diarrhea, nasogastric suction, overuse of lactulose, and drains.

Symptoms include anorexia, muscle weakness and cramps, nausea, vomiting, restlessness, and hyperventilation. Severe symptoms include obtundation, stupor, and coma.

Causes for Rapid Response Activation

Obtundation, stupor, coma.

Actions

INITIAL MEASURES

1. Maintain continuous pulse oximetry.
2. Administer supplemental oxygen to maintain SpO_2 > 95%.
3. Maintain continuous cardiac monitoring/blood pressure measurements.

DIAGNOSTIC WORK-UP

Labs: BMP, magnesium, phosphorus, urea, urine and plasma osmolality, urine sodium, and vasopressin level.

TREATMENT

1. For loss of free water, use 5% dextrose; in patients with hyperglycemia, use half isotonic saline.[2]
2. For sodium gain, use loop diuretics (to cause natriuresis) plus fluid hypotonic to the urine.[2]
3. In acute hypernatremia, correct the serum sodium at an initial rate of 0.5 mmol/L/h (maximum total 12 mmol/L/day).[1,2]
4. Frequently monitor serum sodium level (every 1–2 h initially) during active correction treatment with IV fluids.
5. Perform serial neurologic examinations.
6. Decrease the rate of correction as symptoms of hyponatremia improve.
7. Administer desmopressin (orally or intranasal spray) in patients with central diabetes insipidus.

References

1. Kim SW. Hypernatremia: successful treatment. *Electrolyte Blood Press.* 2006;4(2):66–71.
2. Lindner G, Funk GC. Hypernatremia in critically ill patients. *J Crit Care.* 2013;28. 216.e11–216.e20.

Acute Severe Hyponatremia

Presentation

Acute severe hyponatremia is defined by a serum sodium level < 125 mmol/L for < 48 h.[1] Acute hyponatremia can cause cerebral edema when cells have only a short time to adapt to the hypotonic extracellular environment. The causes of acute severe hyponatremia are:

- Postoperative period (due to high volumes of isotonic fluids)
- Exercise and consumption of hypotonic fluids (competitive marathon runners)
- Psychotic patients with extreme polydipsia
- Medications: haloperidol, thiazide diuretics, IV cyclophosphamide, oxytocin, desmopressin
- Use of irrigants such as glycine or sorbitol during transurethral or hysteroscopic procedures
- 3,4-Methylenedioxymethamphetamine (Ecstasy)[2]

Symptoms of mild-to-moderate hyponatremia include headache, fatigue, nausea, vomiting, disorientation, and confusion. Symptoms of severe hyponatremia are associated with cerebral edema and subsequent brain herniation that will progress to obtundation, seizures, stupor, coma, respiratory arrest, and death.

Causes for Rapid Response Activation

Progressively worsening mental status, seizures, or respiratory failure.

Actions

INITIAL MEASURES

1. Maintain continuous pulse oximetry.
2. Administer supplemental oxygen to maintain SpO_2 > 95%.
3. Maintain continuous cardiac monitoring/blood pressure measurements.

DIAGNOSTIC WORK-UP

Labs: BMP, magnesium, and phosphorus.

TREATMENT

1. For moderate symptoms, use continuous infusion of 3% NaCl 0.5–2 mL/kg/h.[3,4]
2. For severe symptoms, administer bolus 3% NaCl 100 mL over 10 min x 3 repeated doses as needed.[3,4]
3. Minimum recommended correction rate is 4–6 mmol/L/day.[1–3]
4. The limit (not the goal) should be around 10 mmol/L/day for both acute and chronic hyponatremia, and a lower limit of 8 mmol/L/day for patients with high risk of osmotic demyelination syndrome such as initial serum sodium < 105 mmol/L, hypokalemia, alcoholism, malnutrition, or liver disease, for example, liver cirrhosis.[1–3]

5. Frequently monitor serum sodium level (every 1–2 h initially) during active correction treatment with IV fluids.[3]
6. Proactive strategy such as concomitant use of hypertonic saline and desmopressin can be used for patients with SNa <120 mmol/L and high risk of osmotic demyelination syndrome.
7. For treatment of overcorrection of acute hyponatremia, if correction exceeded 6–8 mmol/L/day, start hypotonic fluid such as D5W 3 mL/kg/h IV and desmopressin (DDAVP) 2–4 μg q 6–8 h IV (to stop water diuresis).[3]
8. Manage seizures with parenteral antiepileptic medications.

References

1. Spasovski G, Vanholder R, Allolio B, et al. Clinical practice guideline on diagnosis and treatment of hyponatremia. *Nephrol Dial Transplant.* 2014;29(2):i1–i39.
2. Hoorn EJ, Zietse R. Diagnosis and treatment of hyponatremia: compilation of the guidelines. *J Am Soc Nephrol.* 2017;28(5):1340–1349.
3. Tandukar S, Rondon-Berrios H. Treatment of severe symptomatic hyponatremia. *Physiol Rep.* 2019;7(21), e14265.
4. Verbalis JG, Goldsmith SR, Greenberg A, et al. Diagnosis, evaluation, and treatment of hyponatremia: expert panel recommendations. *Am J Med.* 2013;126(10 Suppl 1):S1–S42.

Acute Severe Hyperkalemia

Presentation

Hyperkalemia may result from excessive intake, decreased excretion, or a shift of potassium from intracellular to extracellular space.

Increased dietary potassium intake is an important cause of hyperkalemia in patients with chronic kidney disease. Total parenteral nutrition and blood transfusions can be other causes of excessive potassium intake.

Decreased potassium excretion occurs in acute or chronic kidney disease. In these conditions, hyperkalemia will usually occur with GFR < 30 mL/min.

Shift of potassium from intracellular to extracellular space can occur in rhabdomyolysis, hemolysis, insulin deficiency, tumor lysis syndrome, metabolic acidosis, or intake of certain drugs, including ACEIs, ARBs, trimethoprim-sulfamethoxazole, succinylcholine, cyclosporine, and tacrolimus.

Hyperkalemia with potassium level > 6.5 mEq/L or EKG changes is a medical emergency. Hyperkalemia is often asymptomatic. Patients may have nonspecific symptoms such as generalized weakness, fatigue, nausea, vomiting, abdominal pain, and diarrhea.[1]

Causes for Rapid Response Activation

Palpitations, syncope, muscle paralysis.

Actions

INITIAL MEASURES

1. Maintain continuous cardiac monitoring.
2. Maintain continuous pulse oximetry.
3. Administer supplemental oxygen in hypoxic patients to maintain SpO_2 > 92% or PaO_2 > 60 mmHg.
4. Discontinue all exogenous sources of potassium.

DIAGNOSTIC WORK-UP

1. 12-Lead and rhythm EKG will show peaked T-waves, shortened QT interval, ST segment depression, prolonged PR interval, widening of QRS duration, loss of P waves, AV conduction delay, and merging of the QRS complex with T wave producing a sine wave pattern and asystole.
2. Labs: CBC, BMP, VBG if acidosis is suspected, urinalysis (assess for glomerulonephritis), urine potassium, urine sodium, urine osmolality, digoxin level if patient is on digitalis medication, creatinine kinase if rhabdomyolysis is suspected, and serum uric acid and phosphorus if tumor lysis is suspected.

TREATMENT

1. Administer calcium gluconate 1.5–3 g IV over 5–10 min to stabilize cardiomyocyte membranes to prevent arrhythmia; onset of action is 1–2 min; duration of action is 30–60 min[2]; calcium has no or minimal effect on the serum level of potassium.
2. Repeat EKG in 5–10 min, and if EKG changes persist, repeat second injection of calcium.[2]
3. Administer regular insulin 10 U IV with 50 mL of 50% dextrose solution (D50) IV to shift potassium into cells; onset of action is 10–20 min; duration of action is 2–6 h; you do not have to administer glucose to patients with hyperglycemia; monitor blood sugars closely.[2]
4. Administer beta-agonist such as albuterol 10–20 mg nebulizer to shift potassium into cells; onset of action is 30 min; duration of action is 4–6 h.[1]
5. Administer furosemide 20–40 mg IV in combination with normal saline infusion in patients with normal kidney function to enhance renal potassium excretion.[2]
6. Administer potassium binders:
   ▪ Sodium polysterene sulfonate (Kayexalate) 15–30 g orally: exchanges sodium for potassium and binds it in the gut; onset of action 2–12 h; duration of action is 4–6 h; avoid in patients with abnormal intestinal function as it may cause intestinal necrosis.[2]
   ▪ Patiromer 8.4 g/packet orally: avoid in patients with abnormal intestinal function, such as severe constipation, bowel obstruction, or severe GI conditions.[3]
7. Start hemodialysis in patients refractory to medical management.
8. In patients with acute kidney injury, proceed with renal ultrasound to assess obstructive uropathy.
9. Assess hydration status and treat dehydration with IV fluids.
10. Monitor serum potassium level closely.

References

1. Best Practices in Managing Hyperkalemia in Chronic Kidney Disease. National Kidney Foundation; 2016. www.kidney.org.
2. Mushiyakh Y, et al. Treatment and pathogenesis of acute hyperkalemia. J Community Hosp Intern Med Perspect. 2011; v1(4).
3. Lederer E, et al. *Hyperkalemia*. Emedicine.medscape.com. Updated: April 09, 2020.

Acute Severe Hypokalemia

Presentation

Severe hypokalemia is defined as serum potassium level < 2.5 mEq/L. Hypokalemia can be due to decreased potassium intake, increased potassium loss (gastrointestinal concerns such as vomiting, diarrhea, or laxative use; renal concerns such as diuretics, renal tubular acidosis, or primary hyperaldosteronism), or transcellular shift (movement of potassium from serum into cells, e.g., due to insulin treatment or thyrotoxicosis).

Symptoms may include palpitations, nausea, vomiting, abdominal cramping, constipation, polyuria, nocturia, weakness, paresis, ascending paralysis, and altered mental status such as psychosis, delirium, hallucinations, and lethargy. On cardiac monitoring, patients may have bradycardia or tachycardia, premature atrial or ventricular beats, or ventricular arrhythmias. On physical examination, patients may have hypotension, hypoventilation, tetany, fasciculations, or decreased or absent tendon reflexes.

Causes for Rapid Response Activation

Severe cardiac arrhythmias, hypotension, progressively worsening neurological findings such as paralysis and progressively worsening mental status.

Actions

INITIAL MEASURES

1. Maintain continuous cardiac monitoring.
2. Maintain continuous pulse oximetry.
3. Administer supplemental oxygen in hypoxic patients to maintain $SpO_2 > 92\%$.

DIAGNOSTIC WORK-UP

1. Labs: BMP, magnesium, phosphorus, digoxin level in patients taking digoxin as hypokalemia can potentiate digitalis-induced arrhythmia, TSH, free T3, free T4, urine electrolytes such as potassium and chloride to differentiate renal from nonrenal causes, urine creatinine (spot urine potassium-to-creatinine ratio > 13 indicates abnormal renal potassium loss), and ABG (to assess for metabolic acidosis or alkalosis or in patients with respiratory failure).
2. EKG: T-wave flattening, inverted T-waves, prominent U waves after T-waves, ST depression, premature atrial contractions, premature ventricular contractions, torsades de pointes, and ventricular fibrillation.

TREATMENT

1. Administer IV potassium for patients with K <2.5 mEq/L; administer no more than 20 mEq of potassium IV to avoid adverse effect on cardiac conduction; combine with oral potassium; recheck potassium level in 3 h.
2. In a symptomatic patient with severe hypokalemia with K <2.5 mEq/L, up to 40 mEq of IV potassium can be administered, however, do so with caution as high doses can cause cardiac complications.
3. If patient has hypomagnesemia, replace magnesium with, magnesium sulfate 2–4 g IV; more than 50% of clinically significant hypokalemia has associated magnesium deficiency, which is most commonly observed in patients using loop or thiazide diuretics.
4. Administer IVF such as 0.9% normal saline.

Further Reading

1. Kardalas E, Paschou SA, Anagnostis P, et al. Hypokalemia: a clinical update. *Endocr Connect.* 2018;7(4):R135–R146.

CHAPTER 6

Hematologic Emergencies

Acute Blood Transfusion Reaction—Febrile Nonhemolytic Reaction

Presentation

Febrile nonhemolytic reaction is a common blood transfusion reaction (1%–35%) and is defined as a temperature $\geq 100.4°F$ or an increase of 1.8°F from pretransfusion value within 24h after a transfusion.[1] Fever may be accompanied by headache, nausea, myalgias, chills, and rigors. This reaction most commonly occurs in patients with multiple prior transfusions and in pregnant patients. Release of cytokines and antibody-mediated endogenous pyrogens from donor's white blood cells leads to development of this reaction.[2]

Causes for Rapid Response Activation

Staff member has significant concern about the patient's condition.

Actions

INITIAL MEASURES

1. Maintain continuous pulse oximetry.
2. Administer supplemental oxygen to maintain $SpO_2 > 95\%$.
3. Maintain continuous cardiac, blood pressure and urine output monitoring, as fever could be the first sign of acute hemolytic reaction, bacterial contamination, or transfusion-related acute lung injury.
4. Stop transfusion.

DIAGNOSTIC WORK-UP

1. Perform a clerical check (patient's ID/blood compatibility label) to determine whether the patient received a correct unit.[2,3]
2. Notify blood bank.[2,3]
3. Perform visual inspection of patient's anticoagulated venous blood; if after centrifugation, patient's plasma has red discoloration (normal plasma is yellow or straw colored), then patient has hemoglobinemia consistent with acute hemolytic reaction.[2,3]

4. Perform visual inspection of patient's urine; if patient developed red urine during transfusion, centrifuge the urine to distinguish between hemoglobinuria and hematuria; if after centrifugation of the urine, red blood cells settle at the bottom of the tube, leaving a clear yellow urine supernatant, the red color of the urine is due to hematuria from the urinary tract; if urine sample remains red after centrifugation, then the red color of urine is due to hemoglobinuria due to acute hemolytic reaction.[2,3]

5. To make sure there is no discrepancy between the original (pretransfusion) and repeat (posttransfusion) ABO typing, return to the blood bank:
   - Residual contents of the donor blood unit container for repeat ABO typing of the donor
   - Freshly collected blood sample from the patient for repeat ABO typing of recipient[2,3]

6. Order direct Coombs test (positive in acute hemolytic reaction).[2,3]

7. Order hemolysis labs: haptoglobin (reduced in hemolysis), LDH (elevated in hemolysis), indirect bilirubin (rises 1 h after the onset of acute hemolytic reaction, with a peak at 5–7 h, and returns to baseline 24 h after the onset of hemolysis), and urobilinogen (elevated in hemolysis).[3]

8. Monitor hemoglobin; it decreases in hemolysis.

9. Febrile nonhemolytic reaction is the diagnosis of exclusion; therefore, rule out other causes of fever, such as sepsis (due to bacterially contaminated blood unit), acute hemolytic reaction, transfusion-related acute lung injury, and anaphylactic reaction.

TREATMENT

1. Administer antipyretic such as acetaminophen 325–500 mg orally.[3]

2. If symptoms have resolved, no clerical error has occurred, visual inspection of plasma shows clear plasma, visual inspection of urine shows normal urine color, retyping of donor and recipient red blood cells for ABO/Rh(D) shows concordant results, Coombs test is negative, and hemolysis labs are normal, then you may resume blood transfusion at a slower rate and continue to monitor the patient closely.[2]

3. Leukoreduction, such as removal or filtration of white blood cells from donor blood, has decreased the rates of febrile nonhemolytic reactions.[1]

References

1. Sharma S, Sharma P, Tyler L. Transfusion of blood and blood products: indications and complications. *Am Fam Physician.* 2011;83(6):719–724.
2. Strobel E. Hemolytic transfusion reactions. *Transfus Med Hemother.* 2008;35(5):346–353.
3. Sandler SG, Johnson VV. *Transfusion Reactions;* 2019. Emedcine.medscape.com.

Urticarial Allergic Reaction

Presentation

Urticarial allergic reaction is common (1%–3% of transfusions)[1] and occurs within 4 h after blood transfusion (most commonly platelets and FFP) and manifests with mucocutaneous signs and symptoms only and without airway compromise or cardiovascular collapse. Urticarial reaction occurs as a result of interaction between IgE antibody of basophils or mast cells in the recipient's blood and allergens to foods or medications in the donor's blood. This interaction causes production of histamine and other substances that lead to hypersensitivity reaction.[2]

Symptoms include generalized flushing, urticaria, pruritus, periorbital/conjunctival erythema, edema and pruritus. Sometimes edema of lips, tongue, and uvula may occur.

Causes for Rapid Response Activation

Staff member has significant concern about the patient's condition.

Actions

INITIAL MEASURES

1. Maintain continuous pulse oximetry.
2. Administer supplemental oxygen to maintain $SpO_2 > 95\%$.
3. Maintain continuous cardiac monitoring and blood pressure measurements, as urticaria could be the first sign of a more severe allergic reaction.
4. Stop transfusion.

DIAGNOSTIC WORK-UP

Generally no further investigation is indicated.

TREATMENT

1. Administer diphenhydramine 25–50 mg IV.[3]
2. Administer methylprednisolone 100–250 mg IV[4] for severe urticarial reactions.
3. If symptoms resolve within 30 min of treatment, resume blood transfusion at a slower rate and continue to monitor the patient closely.
4. Please note, there is evidence that premedication with antihistamines before a transfusion is of no benefit.[5] Use of glucocorticoids for prevention of allergic transfusion reaction has not been studied.[5]

References

1. Sharma S, Sharma P, Tyler L. Transfusion of blood and blood products: indications and complications. *Am Fam Physician.* 2011;83(6):719–724.
2. Hirayama F. Current understanding of allergic transfusion reactions: incidence, pathogenesis, laboratory tests, prevention and treatment. *Br J Haematol.* 2013;160(4):434–444.
3. *Diphenhydramine.* Reference.medscape.com.
4. *Methylprednisolone.* Reference.medscape.com.
5. Savage WJ, Tobian A, Savage JH. Scratching the surface of allergic transfusion reactions. *Transfusion.* 2013;53(6):1361–1371.

Acute Blood Transfusion Reaction—Transfusion Associated Circulatory Overload (TACO)

Presentation

Transfusion associated circulatory overload (TACO) is a common (1%) transfusion reaction. Definition of TACO requires at least one defined criterion with onset up to 12 h after transfusion and a total of three or more criteria, including a pulmonary component, such as respiratory distress or pulmonary edema based on either chest imaging or clinical examination; cardiovascular changes (tachycardia, hypertension, widened pulse pressure, elevated JVP); fluid overload (positive fluid balance, weight gain); or relevant biomarkers (elevated BNP).[1]

Patients with congestive heart failure, renal failure, pulmonary disease, severe anemia, hypoalbuminemia, or advanced age (> 70 years old) are at high risk for fluid overload.

Symptoms may include cough, dyspnea, wheezing, and orthopnea. On physical examination, patients may have hypoxia, tachypnea, tachycardia, elevated blood pressures, distended neck veins, crackles and wheezing on lung auscultation, and peripheral edema.[2]

Causes for Rapid Response Activation

Progressively worsening dyspnea, hypoxia, cyanosis, tachypnea, tachycardia.

Actions

1. Maintain continuous pulse oximetry.
2. Administer supplemental oxygen to maintain $SpO_2 > 95\%$.
3. Maintain continuous cardiac monitoring and blood pressure measurements.
4. Stop the blood transfusion.
5. Move the patient to an upright position.

DIAGNOSTIC WORK-UP

1. Labs: BNP (elevated).[2]
2. Chest X-ray will show bilateral infiltrates consistent with pulmonary vessel engorgement, pulmonary edema, pleural effusions, and cardiomegaly.[2]

TREATMENT

1. Furosemide IV will lead to rapid and significant improvement.[2]
2. If patient requires additional transfusions of RBCs, transfuse lower volumes and a slower rate of 1 mL/kg/h; if possible, select concentrated CPDA-1-anticoagulated red cells with hematocrit 80%–85%.[3]

References

1. Wiersum-Osselton JC, Whitaker B, Grey S, et al. Revised international surveillance case definition of transfusion-associated circulatory overload: a classification agreement validation study. *Lancet Haematol.* 2019;6(7):E350–E358.
2. Semple JW, Rebetz J, Kapur R. Transfusion-associated circulatory overload and transfusion-related acute lung injury. *Blood.* 2019;133(17):1840–1853.
3. Sharma S, Sharma P, Tyler L. Transfusion of blood and blood products: indications and complications. *Am Fam Physician.* 2011;83(6):719–724.

Acute Blood Transfusion Reaction—Transfusion-Related Acute Lung Injury (TRALI)

Presentation

TRALI is a life-threatening complication of transfusion. Antineutrophil cytoplasmic antibodies or anti-HLA antibodies cause noncardiogenic pulmonary edema without circulatory fluid overload.[1] The current incidence is estimated to be 1 in 5000 units of transfused blood.[2] There are no known risk factors to identify patients at risk. All plasma-containing blood products may cause TRALI. It is clinically indistinguishable from acute respiratory distress syndrome (ARDS).

Patients usually develop acute dyspnea and hypoxia within first 6 h of transfusion.[3] Patients may also have fever, tachycardia, and hypotension. Intubated patients may have froth in the endotracheal tube.[2] Mortality rate is 5%–10%.[4] With supportive care, most patients recover within 96 h without permanent sequelae.[4]

Causes for Rapid Response Activation

Worsening dyspnea, cyanosis, hypoxia, tachycardia, hypotension.

Actions

INITIAL MEASURES

1. Stop the blood transfusion immediately.
2. Maintain continuous pulse oximetry.
3. Use high flow oxygen to maintain $SpO_2 > 95\%$.
4. Maintain continuous cardiac monitoring and blood pressure measurements.
5. Request blood bank to quarantine other units from the same donor.[2]

DIAGNOSTIC WORK-UP

TRALI is a clinical diagnosis.
1. Labs: ABG, CBC (will assess acute leukopenia),[2] BNP will help to distinguish cardiogenic pulmonary edema due to circulatory fluid overload from noncardiogenic pulmonary edema due to TRALI.
2. Chest X-ray will assess for bilateral patchy infiltrates consistent with pulmonary edema, which may rapidly develop into complete "white out" very similar to ARDS.[5]
3. Echocardiography may be helpful in distinguishing TRALI and TACO.

TREATMENT

1. Administer fluids conservatively.
2. Use prone positioning for 12–16 h a day to improve gas exchange by decreased V/Q mismatch, decreased lung compression from heart and abdominal organs, and improved drainage of pulmonary secretions.[6]
3. The majority of patients will require intubation and lung-protective mechanical ventilation:
   - Mode: assist control or volume assist
   - Inspiratory to expiratory (I/E) ratio of 1:1 to 1:3
   - RR: 20–35 breaths per minute, usually 20–22 breaths per minute
   - Lower tidal volume: 6 mL/kg of predicted body weight:
   Male: PBW (kg) = 50 + 2.3 (height(in) − 60)
   Female: PBW (kg) = 45.5 + 2.3 (height(in) − 60)
   - Higher PEEP: start at 12 cm of H_2O; may increase up to 28–30 cm of H_2O
   - Plateau airway pressure $\leq 30\,cmH_2O$ to avoid barotrauma[7]
4. Monitoring parameters:
   - Arterial pH of 7.3–7.45
   - SpO_2 of 88%–95%
   - PaO_2 of 55–80 mmHg
   - Plateau pressure $\leq 30\,cmH_2O$[7]
5. There is no role for diuretics or corticosteroids.[5]
6. No special blood product is required for subsequent transfusion of a patient who has developed TRALI.[2]

References

1. Vamvakas EC, Blajchman MA. Transfusion-related mortality: the ongoing risks of allogeneic blood transfusion and the available strategies for their prevention. *Blood.* 2009;113(15):3406–3417.
2. Toy P, Lowell C. TRALI – definition, mechanisms, incidence and clinical relevance. *Best Pract Res Clin Anaesthesiol.* 2007;21(2):183–193.
3. Sharma S, Sharma P, Tyler L. Transfusion of blood and blood products: indications and complications. *Am Fam Physician.* 2011;83(6):719–724.
4. Popovsky MA, Westhoff CM, Bracey A, et al, American Association of Blood Banks. *Guidelines for the Management of Transfusion Related Acute Lung Injury*; 2003. Wrh.on.ca.
5. Petraszko T, Canadian Blood Services. *Transfusion-Related Acute Lung Injury (TRALI)*; 2019. Professionaleducation.blood.ca.
6. Hadaya J, Benharash P. Prone positioning for acute respiratory distress syndrome (ARDS). *JAMA.* 2020;324(13):1361.
7. Saguil A, Fargo M. Acute respiratory distress syndrome: diagnosis and management. *Am Fam Physician.* 2020;101(12):730–738.

Acute Blood Transfusion Reaction—Anaphylactic Reaction

Presentation

Patients with anaphylactic reaction to blood transfusion have been sensitized to the antigens in the donor unit, such as IgA, anti-HLA antibodies, or anticomplement antibodies.[1] Incidence is one in 20,000–50,000 transfusions.[1] Reaction usually begins within 1–45 min after the start of the transfusion. Symptoms include flushing, pruritus, hives, nausea, vomiting, diarrhea, abdominal pain, angioedema, stridor due to laryngeal edema, wheezing due to bronchospasm, dizziness, and hypotension.

Causes for Rapid Response Activation

Progressively worsening dyspnea, stridor, tachycardia, hypotension, syncope.

Actions

INITIAL MEASURES

1. Stop the blood transfusion immediately.
2. Maintain continuous pulse oximetry.
3. Administer supplemental oxygen to maintain $SpO_2 > 95\%$, usually 8–10 L/min.
4. Maintain continuous cardiac monitoring/blood pressure measurements.
5. Place patient supine.

DIAGNOSTIC WORK-UP

Anti-IgA in a pretransfusion sample of the recipient's serum or plasma establishes the diagnosis; if this test is not available, screen for IgA deficiency; the presence of IgA in the recipient's pretransfusion sample excludes the diagnosis of a class-specific IgA/anti-IgA reaction.

TREATMENT[2]

1. Administer epinephrine 0.3–0.5 mL of a 1:1000 aqueous solution subcutaneously or intramuscularly, usually into the upper arm; repeat the dose two or three times at 10–15 min intervals.
2. In patient with severe hypotension in whom subcutaneous epinephrine is ineffective, start continuous infusion of epinephrine 1:10,000 aqueous solution at 1 μg/min and titrate up to 10 μg/min.
3. Patients taking β-blockers may be refractory to epinephrine; in this case, glucagon 1 mg IV bolus may be useful; this treatment can be followed by a continuous infusion of glucagon 1–5 mg/h.

4. Start aggressive fluid resuscitation.
5. Vasopressors for the patients refractory to volume replacement:
   - Dopamine at 2–20 µg/kg/min
6. Administer continuous nebulized albuterol 10–15 mg for 1 h for patients with bronchospasm.
7. Administer diphenhydramine 25–50 mg IV.
8. Administer cimetidine 4 mg/kg IV.
9. Administer hydrocortisone 100–250 mg IV.

References

1. Sharma S, Sharma P, Tyler L. Transfusion of blood and blood products: indications and complications. *Am Fam Physician.* 2011;83(6):719–724.
2. Tang AW. A practical guide to anaphylaxis. *Am Fam Physician.* 2003;68(7):1325–1333.

Acute Blood Transfusion Reaction—Acute Hemolytic Reaction

Presentation

Acute hemolytic reactions occur within the first 24 h of transfusion and are usually caused by transfusion of incompatible blood cells. The incidence rate is 1 in 70,000 RBC transfusions.[1] May be immune-mediated or nonimmune-mediated. Immune-mediated reactions could cause severe hemolysis due to anti-A, anti-B, or anti-AB antibodies or mild hemolysis due to IgG, Rh, or Kell or Duffy antibodies.[2] These antibodies are produced after immunization through a previous transfusion or pregnancy.

Early signs may include fever, chills, rigors, burning sensation at the infusion site, flushing, nausea, vomiting, abdominal pain, chest pain, back pain, dyspnea, wheezing, red-colored urine, and oliguria/anuria. Later symptoms may include diffuse bleeding due to DIC (disseminated intravascular coagulation), hypotension, and worsening renal failure requiring hemodialysis.[1]

Causes for Rapid Response Activation

Chest pain, progressively worsening dyspnea, tachypnea, tachycardia, hypotension.

Actions

INITIAL MEASURES

1. Maintain continuous pulse oximetry.
2. Administer supplemental oxygen to maintain $SpO_2 > 95\%$.
3. Assure continuous cardiac monitoring, blood pressure measurements and monitoring of urine output.
4. Immediately stop transfusion.

DIAGNOSTIC WORK-UP

1. Perform a clerical check (patient's ID/blood compatibility label) to determine whether the patient received a correct unit.[1,3]
2. Notify blood bank.[1,3]
3. Perform visual inspection of patient's anticoagulated venous blood; if after centrifugation, patient's plasma has red discoloration (normal plasma is yellow or straw colored), then patient has hemoglobinemia consistent with acute hemolytic reaction.[1,3]

4. Perform visual inspection of patient's urine; if patient developed red urine during transfusion, centrifuge the urine to distinguish between hemoglobinuria and hematuria; if after centrifugation of the urine, red blood cells settle at the bottom of the tube, leaving a clear yellow urine supernatant, the red color of the urine is due to hematuria from the urinary tract; if urine sample remains red after centrifugation, then the red color of the urine is due to hemoglobinuria due to acute hemolytic reaction.[1,3]

5. To make sure there is no discrepancy between the original (pretransfusion) and repeat (posttransfusion) ABO typing, return to the blood bank:
   - Residual contents of the donor blood unit container for repeat ABO typing of the donor
   - Freshly collected blood sample from the patient for repeat ABO typing of recipient[1,3]

6. Order direct Coombs test (positive in acute hemolytic reaction).[1,3]

7. Order hemolysis labs: haptoglobin (reduced in hemolysis), LDH (elevated in hemolysis), indirect bilirubin (rises 1 h after the onset of acute hemolytic reaction, with a peak at 5–7 h and returns to baseline 24 h after the onset of hemolysis), and urobilinogen (elevated in hemolysis).[3]

8. Peripheral blood smear will show helmet cells, bite cells, or spherocytes.

9. Monitor CBC; hemoglobin and hematocrit will decrease in hemolysis.

10. Monitor coagulations studies, such as INR (increased), PT (prolonged), aPTT (prolonged), fibrinogen (decreased), antithrombin, D-dimer (increased), and fibrin degradation products (elevated) to assess the severity of DIC.

11. Monitor BMP to assess renal failure and electrolyte abnormalities.

12. Monitor ABG for acidosis.

TREATMENT

1. Start aggressive IVF hydration with 0.9% sodium chloride as a 500 mL/h bolus, followed by 100–150 mL/h; use vital signs (heart rate, blood pressure, respiratory rate, oxygen saturation) and urine output (1 mL/kg/h is a goal urine output) to guide fluid resuscitation.[1,3]

2. Consider dopamine 2–5 μg/kg/min to improve renal perfusion (inconsistent evidence).[1]

3. Consider furosemide to improve renal output; however, if no response occurs within 1–2 h, consult nephrologist for consideration of hemodialysis.[1]

4. Administer FFP, fibrinogen, and platelets for treatment of DIC.[1]

5. Ensure adequate airway.

6. Consult hematologist early in the course of rapid response.

References

1. Strobel E. Hemolytic transfusion reactions. *Transfus Med Hemother.* 2008;35(5):346–353.
2. Harewood J, Ramsey A, Master SR. *Hemolytic Transfusion Reaction.* StatPearls Publishing; 2020.
3. Sandler SG, Johnson VV. *Transfusion Reactions*; 2019. Emedcine.medscape.com.

Acute Heparin-Induced Thrombocytopenia (HIT)

Presentation

Heparin-induced thrombocytopenia is a prothrombotic adverse drug reaction and usually occurs 4–10 days after exposure to heparin.[1] The most commonly used pharmacological VTE prophylaxes in hospitalized patients are unfractionated heparin (UFH) and low-molecular-weight heparin (LMWH). HIT is usually mediated by immunoglobulin G antibodies against complexes of platelet factor 4 (PF4) and heparin.[2] Incidence of heparin-induced thrombocytopenia is about 0.2% in all heparin-exposed patients.[3]

HIT is suspected when a patient receiving a heparin product has a decrease in the platelet count, particularly if the decrease is > 50% of the baseline count, even if the platelet count nadir is $> 150 \times 10^9/L$.[4]

Before initiation of heparin products, all patients should have their baseline platelet count checked. According to the American Society of Hematology (ASH),[5] when HIT is suspected:

- Calculate 4T's score (thrombocytopenia, timing of platelet count fall, thrombosis or other sequelae, and other causes of thrombocytopenia).
- If 4T's score is ≤3, HIT probability is low; do not order HIT lab testing and continue heparin.
- If 4T's score is ≥4, HIT probability is intermediate/high; discontinue heparin, start nonheparin anticoagulant, and obtain immunoassay.
- If immunoassay is negative, discontinue nonheparin anticoagulation and resume heparin.
- If immunoassay is positive, obtain functional assay.
- If functional assay is negative, discontinue nonheparin anticoagulation and resume heparin.
- If functional assay is positive, continue avoidance of heparin and follow guidelines on treatment of acute HIT.

Symptoms of acute HIT include skin lesions at heparin injection sites. Patients may develop systemic reactions such as fever, chills, dyspnea, or chest pain after infusion of IV bolus of heparin. About 30%–50% of HIT cases are complicated by venous (more common) or arterial (less common) thromboembolism.[5]

Causes for Rapid Response Activation

Progressively worsening dyspnea, chest pain, tachycardia, tachypnea, hypotension.

Actions

INITIAL MEASURES

Discontinue all heparin products, including heparin flushes of IV catheters.

DIAGNOSTIC WORK-UP

1. Order immunoassay to detect antibodies against heparin and platelet factor 4 (PF 4) complexes.
2. Functional assay measures the platelet-activating capacity of PF4 and heparin-antibody complexes and is more specific than immunoassay; however, it has a long turnaround time and is not available at all hospitals.
3. Order bilateral lower extremity Doppler ultrasonography to screen for asymptomatic proximal deep vein thrombosis (DVT).
4. Order upper extremity Doppler ultrasonography in the limb with the central venous catheter to screen for asymptomatic DVT.
5. Order CT angiogram of chest if there is a suspicion of pulmonary embolism.

TREATMENT[5]

1. Administer nonheparin anticoagulant in clinically stable patients with average risk of bleeding:
   - Fondaparinux
     - 5mg SC once daily (<50kg)
     - 7.5 mg SC daily (50–100 kg)
     - 10 mg SC daily (>100 kg)
   - Continue until platelet count recovery (a platelet count of $\geq 150 \times 10^9/L$) in HIT without thrombosis and for 3–6 m in HIT with thrombosis.
   - Administer direct oral anticoagulant (DOAC):
     - Rivaroxaban 15 mg twice per day until platelet count recovery (a platelet count of $\geq 150 \times 10^9/L$) in HIT without thrombosis
     - Rivaroxaban 15 mg twice per day for 3 weeks, followed by 20 mg once per day for 3–6 m in HIT with thrombosis
     - Apixaban 5 mg twice per day until platelet count recovery (a platelet count of $\geq 150 \times 10^9/L$) in HIT without thrombosis
     - Apixaban 10 mg twice per day for 1 week, then 5 mg twice per day for 3–6 m in HIT with thrombosis
2. Administer nonheparin anticoagulant in critically ill patients with higher risk of bleeding:
   - Argatroban continuous infusion 2 µg/kg/min; administer 0.5–1.2 µg/kg/min in patients with liver disease, CHF, anasarca, or postcardiac surgery.
   - Bivalirudin 0.15 mg/kg/h; dose reduction will be required for patients with liver or renal dysfunction.
   - Continue until platelet count recovery (a platelet count of $\geq 150 \times 10^9/L$) in HIT without thrombosis.
3. In patients taking warfarin:
   - Discontinue warfarin.
   - Administer vitamin K IV in addition to a nonheparin anticoagulant.
   - May restart warfarin after platelet count recovery (a platelet count of $\geq 150 \times 10^9/L$).
4. May consider administering platelet transfusion:
   - Average bleeding risk: the ASH guideline panel suggests against routine platelet transfusion.
   - High bleeding risk or active bleeding: platelet transfusion may be an option.
5. The ASH guideline panel recommends against routine insertion of an inferior vena cava (IVC) filter.

References

1. Warkentin TE, Greinacher A. Heparin-induced thrombocytopenia: recognition, treatment, and prevention: the Seventh ACCP Conference on Antithrombotic and Thrombolytic Therapy. *Chest.* 2004;126(3):311S–337S.
2. Amiral J, Bridey F, Dreyfus M, et al. Platelet factor 4 complexed to heparin is the target for antibodies generated in heparin-induced thrombocytopenia. *Thromb Haemost.* 1992;68(1):95–96.
3. Smythe MA, Koerber JM, Mattson JC. The incidence of recognized heparin-induced thrombocytopenia in a large, tertiary care teaching hospital. *Chest.* 2007;131(6):1644–1649.
4. Sankar E. *Heparin Induced Thrombocytopenia*; 2019. Emedicine.medscpae.com.
5. Cuker A, Arepally GM, Chong BH, et al. American Society of Hematology 2018 guidelines for management of venous thromboembolism: heparin-induced thrombocytopenia. *Blood Adv.* 2018;2(22):3360–3392.

Disseminated Intravascular Coagulation (DIC)

Presentation

DIC is usually a complication of other serious underlying illnesses. DIC is due to systemic activation of blood coagulation that results in fibrin deposition leading to thromboses in microvasculature of different organs and resulting in multiorgan failure. Simultaneously, consumption of platelets and clotting factors leads to life-threatening bleeding.

Conditions that activate intravascular blood coagulation include sepsis, pancreatitis, liver disease, vascular abnormalities, malignancy, severe transfusion reactions, transplant rejections, and other conditions.

In addition to the symptoms of the underlying condition causing DIC, patients may develop petechiae, ecchymosis, gingival bleeding, oozing from IV lines and catheters, and gastrointestinal bleeding. Postoperative patients may have oozing from surgical incisions, drains, and tracheostomies.[1]

Causes for Rapid Response Activation

Severe dyspnea or hemoptysis in patients with pulmonary involvement, worsening mental status (stupor, coma), or focal neurologic deficits in patients with neurologic involvement and tachycardia/hypotension due to life-threatening hemorrhage.

Actions

INITIAL MEASURES

1. Maintain continuous pulse oximetry
2. Administer supplemental oxygen to maintain $SpO_2 > 92\%$
3. Maintain continuous cardiac monitoring

DIAGNOSTIC WORK-UP

Labs: CBC (low hemoglobin, thrombocytopenia), peripheral smear (schistocytes), prolonged coagulation times (PT, aPTT), elevated fibrin degradation products, elevated D-dimer, and low fibrinogen level.

TREATMENT

1. Treat underlying disease causing DIC; for example, treat sepsis with appropriate antibiotics, control the source of infection (e.g., drain liver abscess), and treat malignancy with chemotherapy; the only exception is massive bleeding type of DIC.
2. Start IVF resuscitation to correct hypovolemia.
3. Transfuse packed red blood cells when indicated to treat anemia.

4. Transfuse 6–8 platelet concentrates or single apheresis unit if:
   - Platelets $\leq 20 \times 10^9$/L and no bleeding
   - Platelet count $\leq 50 \times 10^9$/L and bleeding
   - Early postoperative phase
   - Invasive procedure planned
   - At risk for bleeding complications[1-3]
5. Transfuse FFP 15–30 mL/kg if:
   - Active bleeding is occurring
   - Patient is in early postoperative phase
   - Invasive procedure is planned
   - Patient is at risk for bleeding complications[1-3]
   - In patients with fluid overload, consider prothrombin complex concentrate instead of FFP; however, prothrombin complex concentrate lacks some factors, such as factor V
6. Administer fibrinogen concentrate 3 g or cryoprecipitate in severe hypofibrinogenemia <1 g/dL that persists despite FFP replacement.[2]
7. Monitor response to blood therapy clinically and with serial CBC and coagulation parameters.

References

1. Levi M, Nagalla S. *Disseminated Intravascular Coagulopathy Treatment and Management.* Emedicine. medscape.com. Updated: December 06, 2020.
2. Levi M, Toh CH, Thachil J, Watson HG. Guidelines for the diagnosis and management of intravascular disseminated coagulation. British committee for standards in haematology. *Br J Haematol.* 2009;145(1):24–33.
3. Wada H, Matsumoto T, Yamashita Y. Diagnosis and treatment of disseminated intravascular coagulation (DIC) according to four DIC guidelines. *J Intensive Care.* 2014;2(1):15.

Acute Chest Syndrome in Sickle Cell Disease

Presentation

Acute chest syndrome is a leading cause of mortality in patients with sickle cell disease.[1] Acute chest syndrome is defined as a new pulmonary infiltrate on plain chest film, accompanied by fever and respiratory symptoms.[2] The prevalence of sickle cell disease is low and is estimated to affect 100,000 people in the United States.[2] Risk factors for acute chest syndrome include smoking, asthma, recent trauma, surgery, and anesthesia.

Symptoms and signs include fever, chest pain, pain in arms/legs, cough, wheezing, dyspnea, and tachypnea. In a small subset of adults, rapidly progressive acute chest syndrome may develop, causing acute kidney injury, acute liver failure, neurologic deterioration, and multiorgan failure.

Causes for Rapid Response Activation

Acute respiratory failure with severe hypoxia due to noncardiogenic pulmonary edema, altered mental status.

Actions

INITIAL MEASURES

1. Continuous pulse oximetry may be inaccurate; CO-oximetry measures oxygen saturation more accurately in patients with sickle cell disease.
2. Administer supplemental oxygen to maintain $SpO_2 > 92\%$.
3. Maintain continuous cardiac monitoring.

DIAGNOSTIC WORK-UP

1. Labs: CBC with differential (anemia; thrombocytopenia is an independent risk factor for respiratory failure), ABG in patients with worsening respiratory failure (A-a gradient is the best predictor of clinical severity),[3] and blood and sputum cultures in febrile patients; also consider a troponin test.
2. Order EKG.
3. Order AP and lateral chest X-ray to assess for new pulmonary infiltrate, multiple lobes may be involved, and pleural effusions.
4. Order CT angiogram of chest when pulmonary embolism is suspected.

TREATMENT

1. Administer oxygen therapy.
2. Administer incentive spirometry, 10 maximal breaths every 2 h, while patient is awake to prevent hypoventilation or atelectasis.

3. Administer inhaled bronchodilators, for example, continuous albuterol nebulization at 10 mg/h,[4] especially in patients with asthma.

4. Administer IV fluids to address hypovolemia; usually 1.5 times maintenance fluids of D5 in 1/2 normal saline[5] for the first 24–48 h; decrease the rate when patient has improved oral intake; avoid overhydration to prevent pulmonary edema.

5. Assure adequate pain control with parenteral opioids; consider patient-controlled analgesia; avoid oversedation to prevent hypoxia and hypoventilation.

6. Administer transfused packed red blood cells to the goal of Hg of 10 g/dL to increase oxygen affinity of blood:
   - At first sign of hypoxia
   - Hg 10%–20% below baseline
   - Hg < 5 g/dL
   - Clinical or radiographic deterioration
   - Exchange transfusion delayed

7. Start exchange transfusion by automated erythrocytapheresis of large amounts of blood up to 6–8 units[6] to decrease hemoglobin S burden for patients with moderate or severe acute chest pain syndrome when:
   - Pulmonary infiltrates involve > 1 lobe
   - Oxygen requirement > 4 L via nasal cannula
   - There are signs of clinical deterioration or severe hypoxia[7]

8. Target therapeutic end-points for erythrocytapheresis:
   - Hemoglobin S < 30%
   - Hemoglobin 10 g/dL[7]

9. Administer broad-spectrum IV antibiotics, with coverage of atypical microorganisms, as they are common in sickle cell disease, for febrile patients[5]:
   - Cefotaxime 2 g IV q 6–8 h[8] and azithromycin 500 mg IV[9] once daily for 7–10 days
   - Moxifloxacin 400 mg IV[10] for 7 days

10. Assure mechanical and pharmacological VTE prophylaxis.

11. Cases refractory to treatment may need intubation and mechanical ventilation and pulmonology consultation for bronchoscopy and bronchoalveolar lavage.

References

1. Platt OS, Brambilla DJ, Rosse WF, et al. Mortality is sickle cell disease. Life expectancy and risk factors for early death. *N Engl J Med.* 1994;330(23):1639.
2. Ballas SK, Lieff S, Benjamin LJ, et al. Definitions of the phenotypic manifestations of sickle cell disease. *Am J Hematol.* 2010;85(1):6.
3. Emre U, Miller ST, Rao SP, et al. Alveolar-arterial oxygen gradient in acute chest syndrome of sickle cell disease. *J Pediatr.* 1993;123:272–275.
4. *Albuterol.* Reference.medscape.com.
5. Vichinsky EP, Neumayr LD, Earles AN, et al. Causes and outcomes of the acute chest syndrome in sickle cell disease. *N Engl J Med.* 2000;342:1855–1865.
6. Verduzco LA, Nathan DG. Sickle cell disease and stroke. *Blood.* 2009;114(25):5117.
7. Friend A, Girzadas D. *Acute Chest Syndrome.* StatPearls Publishing; 2020.
8. *Cefotaxime.* Reference.medscape.com.
9. *Azithromycin.* Reference.medscape.com.
10. *Moxifloxacin.* Reference.medscape.com.

Acute Immune Thrombocytopenia (ITP)

Presentation

Immune thrombocytopenia is a rare blood disorder characterized by normal bone marrow and occurs due to acquired autoimmune destruction of platelets. Spontaneous bleeding—such as petechiae (small purple dots); purpura (bruises); and mucosal, intracranial, gastrointestinal, and genitourinary bleeding—is more likely to occur in patients with platelet counts less than 5×10^9/L, and is a hematologic emergency.[1] Patients with intracranial hemorrhage may have blurry vision, headache, and altered mental status.

Causes for Rapid Response Activation

Altered mental status (e.g., somnolence, loss of consciousness), focal neurological symptoms due to intracranial bleeding, hypertension and bradycardia due to increased intracranial pressure, any type of spontaneous bleeding.

Actions

INITIAL MEASURES

1. Maintain continuous pulse oximetry.
2. Administer supplemental oxygen to maintain $SpO_2 > 92\%$.
3. Maintain continuous cardiac monitoring.
4. Consult hematologist early in the course of rapid response.
5. Consult neurosurgeon for patients with intracranial hemorrhage.

DIAGNOSTIC WORK-UP

1. Labs: CBC (usually isolated thrombocytopenia, low hemoglobin due to hemorrhage), peripheral smear (normal RBC and WBC morphology, sometimes large platelets), coagulation studies (usually normal), and pregnancy test.
2. Order type and screen.
3. Order noncontrast CT scan of the head if concerned about intracranial hemorrhage.
4. Order CT scan or MRI if internal bleeding is present.
5. Bone marrow biopsy will show normal bone marrow cells; consideration of bone marrow biopsy is recommended for thrombocytopenic adults > 60 years old and for all adults before initiation of steroid treatment.[2]

TREATMENT

1. Administer IV fluids to patients with hypovolemia.
2. Administer high dose of glucocorticoids such as dexamethasone 40 mg IV per day for 4 days; will raise platelets within 1–2 days[3]; monitor for hypertension and hyperglycemia; followed by oral prednisone taper ≤6 weeks.
3. Administer intravenous immunoglobulin single dose of 1 g/kg[3]; the dose may be repeated if necessary.
4. Platelet transfusion is indicated for:
   - Platelet count $< 50 \times 10^9$/L and bleeding, including significant mucous membrane bleeding
   - Platelet count < 20–30×10^9/L
   - Patients with risk factors for bleeding (hypertension, peptic ulcer disease)[3,4]
5. Transfuse 6–8 U of platelet concentrate (1 U of platelets will increase platelet count of a 70-kg adult by 5–10×10^9/L); transfuse immediately after IVIG infusion to increase platelet survival.[3,4]
6. Transfuse packed red blood cells when indicated to treat anemia.
7. Four weekly IV infusions of rituximab at a dose of 375 mg/m² showed a response rate of up to 60%.[5]

References

1. Gauer RL, Braun MM. Thrombocytopenia. *Am Fam Physician.* 2012;85(6):612–622.
2. Jubelirer SJ, Harpold R. The role of bone marrow examination in the diagnosis of immune thrombocytopenic purpura: case series and literature review. *Clin Appl Thromb Hemost.* 2002;8(1):73–76.
3. Neunert C, Terrell DR, et al. American Society of Hematology guidelines for immune thrombocytopenia. *Blood Adv.* 2019;3(23):3829–3866.
4. Silverman MA, Shlamovitz GZ, et al. *Immune Thrombocytopenia (ITP) in Emergency Medicine.* Medscape.com. Updated: December 14, 2019.
5. Lucchini E, Zaja F, Bussel J. Rituximab in the treatment of immune thrombocytopenia: what is the role of this agent in 2019? *Haematologica.* 2019;104:1124–1135.

Thrombotic Thrombocytopenic Purpura (TTP)

Presentation

TTP is a rare blood disorder characterized by microthrombi in small blood vessels, resulting in a low platelet count. TTP occurs due to antibodies against ADAMTS-13 (a disintegrin and metalloproteinase with a thrombospondin type 1 motif member 13)—a protein that cleaves von Willebrand factor, which causes platelet aggregation and thromboses in microvasculature of brain, kidneys, and heart, causing their ischemia and injury.[1]

About 20%–30% of patients will have the pentad of fever, microangiopathic hemolytic anemia (fatigue, pallor, jaundice), thrombocytopenic purpura (petechiae), neurologic abnormalities, and renal disease.[1] If untreated, this condition has high mortality.

Causes for Rapid Response Activation

Acute mental state changes, seizure, stroke-like symptoms such as aphasia, visual changes, paresthesias, hemiplegia, or any type of severe bleeding.

Actions

INITIAL MEASURES

1. Maintain continuous pulse oximetry.
2. Administer supplemental oxygen to maintain $SpO_2 > 92\%$.
3. Maintain continuous cardiac monitoring.
4. Consult hematologist early in the course of rapid response.
5. Consult neurosurgeon for patients with intracranial hemorrhage.
6. Consult nephrologist if acute kidney injury requires hemodialysis.

DIAGNOSTIC WORK-UP

1. Labs: CBC (thrombocytopenia, low hemoglobin due to hemorrhage, increased reticulocyte count), peripheral blood smear (schistocytes due to hemolysis), coagulation studies (normal), CMP (elevated creatinine, elevated indirect/unconjugated bilirubin due to hemolysis), lactate dehydrogenase (elevated due to hemolysis), haptoglobin (decreased due to hemolysis), urinalysis (proteinuria and hematuria in renal disease), and pregnancy test.
2. Reduced ADAMTS-13 activity ($< 5\%$) and presence of IgG antibodies will confirm diagnosis of TTP[2]; however, test results are not immediately available.
3. Order head CT scan or MRI to rule out infarct or hemorrhage.

TREATMENT

1. Consult surgeon for placement of a central venous line to start apheresis.
2. Start total plasma exchange with solvent/detergent-treated fresh frozen plasma (Octaplas) within 4–8 h to remove autoantibodies against ADAMTS-13; administer 1–5 plasma volumes × 3, then 1 plasma volume/day and continue for a minimum of 2 days after platelet count has been > 150×10^9/L; then stop.[2]
3. If there is a delay in arrangement of plasma exchange, start FFP infusion and monitor for fluid overload; solvent/detergent-treated FFP is preferred over standard FFP to reduce the risk of transfusion-transmitted infection and adverse immune responses such as allergic reactions, anaphylaxis, or central venous catheter thrombosis.[2]
4. Administer methylprednisolone 1 g IV daily for 3 days.[2]
5. Transfuse packed red blood cells when indicated to treat anemia.
6. Administer rituximab 375 mg/m^2 IV weekly for 4 weeks; for patients refractory to plasma exchange and steroid treatment or with neurologic or cardiac involvement,[2] ideally, at least 4 h should elapse between administration of rituximab and plasma exchange.[2]
7. Administer cryosupernatant (fresh frozen plasma that has had the cryoprecipitate removed and is thus depleted of high-molecular-weight von Willebrand multimers) to patients refractory to plasma exchange.[1]
8. For thrombosis prevention, when platelet count > 50×10^9/L, start low-molecular-weight heparin thromboprophylaxis.[2]
9. Avoid platelet transfusions unless life-threatening bleeding, such as central nervous system bleeding, is present.

References

1. Wun T, Nagalla S. *Thrombotic Thrombocytopenic Purpura (TTP) Treatment and Management.* Medscape.com. Updated: May 25, 2021.
2. Scully M, Hunt BJ, et al. Guidelines on the diagnosis and management of thrombotic and thrombocytopenic purpura and other thrombotic microangiopathies. *Br J Haematol.* 2012;158(3):323–335.

Atypical Hemolytic Uremic Syndrome (HUS)

Presentation

HUS is a rare blood disorder characterized by thrombotic microangiopathy. HUS usually presents with hemolytic anemia, thrombocytopenia, and acute kidney injury. It is very uncommon in adults.[1] There are two types of HUS: Shiga-like toxin associated HUS, which usually occurs in children younger than 2–3 years, and non-Shiga-like toxin associated HUS or atypical HUS, which accounts for 5%–10% of HUS cases and usually occurs in adults.[2]

Atypical HUS is due to genetic complement abnormalities and is triggered by infections such as *Streptococcus pneumoniae*, drugs (e.g., quinine; chemotherapy drugs such as cisplatin, bleomycin; antiplatelets such as clopidogrel; oral contraceptives), malignancies (e.g., mucin-producing adenocarcinoma), pregnancy, transplantation and calcineurin inhibitors, and other conditions.[2]

Symptoms include fatigue, irritability, and lethargy. Patient may have headache due to hypertension. Prognosis is poor. Acute kidney injury may progress into end-stage renal disease necessitating dialysis.[3]

Causes for Rapid Response Activation

Worsening altered mental status, such as lethargy and confusion; stroke-like symptoms; seizure.

Actions

INITIAL MEASURES

1. Maintain continuous pulse oximetry.
2. Administer supplemental oxygen to maintain $SpO_2 > 92\%$.
3. Maintain continuous cardiac monitoring.
4. Consult hematologist early in the course of rapid response.
5. Consult neurosurgeon for patients with intracranial hemorrhage.
6. Consult nephrologist if acute kidney injury requires hemodialysis.

DIAGNOSTIC WORK-UP

1. Labs: CBC (decrease hemoglobin, thrombocytopenia), peripheral smear (schistocytes), CMP (elevated creatinine, elevated indirect bilirubin, low albumin), LDH (elevated), haptoglobin (low), urinalysis (proteinuria, hematuria, RBC casts), complement serology testing.
2. Renal ultrasound to rule out obstruction.

TREATMENT

1. Administer IV fluids in the absence of fluid overload.

2. Treat hypertension with vasodilators:
   - Hydralazine 5–10 mg IV q 4 h as needed
3. Transfuse packed red blood cells when Hg < 7 g/dL.
4. Platelet transfusion is contraindicated unless:
   - Severe hemorrhage present
   - Surgical intervention planned[3]
5. Two monoclonal antibodies were approved by the FDA (Federal Drug Administration) as a first-line therapy for confirmed or strongly suspected atypical HUS; these antibodies reduce hemolysis, improve platelet count, and reverse acute kidney injury[4]:
   - Eculizumab[5]
     Doses 1–4: 900 mg IV q week for first 4 weeks, followed by
     Dose 5: 1200 mg IV 1 week later; then
     1200 mg IV q 2 weeks thereafter
   - Ravulizumab
6. Patients without history of appropriate meningococcal vaccination must be immunized with meningococcal vaccines at least 2 weeks before starting treatment with monoclonal antibodies.[6]
7. In unvaccinated patient requiring immediate initiation of eculizumab or ravulizumab:
   - Administer meningococcal vaccine as soon as possible.
   - Provide 2 weeks of antibacterial drug prophylaxis.[6]
8. If unable to use monoclonal antibodies, start plasmapheresis:[3]
   - Plasma exchange at 1.5 plasma volumes per session
   - Daily plasma exchange five times a week for 2 weeks, followed by three times a week for the subsequent 2 weeks.

References

1. Perez-Cruz FG, Villa-Diaz P, Pintado-Delgado MC, et al. Hemolytic uremic syndrome in adults: a case report. *World J Crit Care Med.* 2017;6(2):135–139.
2. Parmar MS. *Hemolytic Uremic Syndrome.* Emedicine.medscape.com. Updated: October 25, 2019.
3. Salvadori M, Bertoni E. Update on hemolytic uremic syndrome: diagnostic and therapeutic recommendations. *World J Nephrol.* 2013;2(3):56–76.
4. Lieberman K. Atypical Hemolytic Uremic Syndrome. NORD National Organization for Rare Disorders; 2016. Rarediseases.org.
5. *Eculizumab.* Reference.medscape.com.
6. *Soliris (eculizumab).* Soliris.net.

CHAPTER 7

Oncologic Emergencies

Tumor Lysis Syndrome

Presentation

Tumor lysis syndrome is a metabolic emergency due to rapid cell lysis and presents as acute kidney failure and severe electrolyte abnormalities such as hyperkalemia, hyperphosphatemia, hyperuricemia, and hypocalcemia. This syndrome is associated with acute leukemias, high-grade lymphomas, or large solid tumors and can occur either spontaneously or within 7 days of cancer treatment initiation. Usually it occurs in association with chemotherapy; however, it can also occur after radiation and biological drugs.[1,2]

Causes for Rapid Response Activation

Severe dyspnea due to fluid overload, syncope, cardiac dysrhythmias, seizure, tetany.

Actions

INITIAL MEASURES

1. Withhold cancer treatment.
2. Maintain continuous pulse oximetry.
3. Administer supplemental oxygen to maintain $SpO_2 > 92\%$.
4. Maintain continuous cardiac monitoring.

DIAGNOSTIC WORK-UP

1. 12-Lead and rhythm EKG.
2. Labs: CBC (leukocytosis, anemia, thrombocytopenia), BMP (elevated potassium and creatinine, low calcium), uric acid (elevated), phosphorus (elevated), LDH (elevated).
3. Serial BMP, uric acid, phosphorus at least q 8 h with rapid laboratory turnover time for at least 48–72 h to monitor response to therapy.

TREATMENT

1. Start aggressive IV hydration in patients without fluid overload. About 4–5 L/d might be needed with goal urine output of about 3L/d.[3]
2. To control hyperuricemia, administer allopurinol 600–900 mg PO daily divided q8–12 h; if patient is unable to take PO, administer allopurinol 200–400 mg/m²/day, as single infusion

or in equally divided doses IV; it is administered to reduce the conversion of nucleic acid byproducts to uric acid in order to prevent urate nephropathy.[3]

3. If allopurinol alone is not sufficient to reduce uric acid level, stop allopurinol and administer rasburicase 0.2 mg/kg IV over 30 min once daily; this treatment works by converting uric acid to water-soluble metabolites; it is contraindicated in G6PD deficiency and pregnancy.[3]

4. Hyperkalemia is treated based on K levels[3]:
   - K 5.0–5.9 mmol/L: Administer Kayexalate 15 g PO; repeat q 4–6 h depending on potassium level; if unable to take PO, administer 30–50 g every 6 h rectally in a retention enema; avoid Kayexalate in patients with constipation, inflammatory bowel disease, or postoperative patients.
   - K ≥ 6 mmol/L: Administer regular insulin 10 U IV followed immediately by 50 mL of 50% glucose (25 g) IV (if blood glucose is < 250 mg/dL) with or without albuterol nebulizer 10–20 mg over 20 min; monitor blood glucose closely.
   - K > 6.5 mmol/L or for patients with EKG changes (marked QRS widening): Administer calcium gluconate 1.5–3 g IV for cardioprotection; if follow-up EKG in 5 min continues to show signs of hyperkalemia, repeat the dose; please note, this is in addition to regular insulin, glucose and albuterol.

5. Hyperphosphatemia is treated with phosphate binders, such as sevelamer hydrochloride (Renagel)[3]:
   - Serum PO_4 > 9 mg/dL: 1600 mg PO q 8 h with meals
   - Serum PO_4 7.5–9 mg/dL: 1200 mg PO q 8 h with meals
   - Serum PO_4 5.5–7.5 mg/dL: 800 mg PO q 8 h with meals

6. To treat hypocalcemia, treat hyperphosphatemia, as hypocalcemia resolves as phosphate levels normalize.

7. If all above therapies fail, consult nephrology for continuous renal-replacement therapy and continue frequent monitoring of electrolytes.

References

1. Higdon ML, Atkinson CJ, Lawrence KV. Oncologic emergencies: recognition and initial management. *Am Fam Physician.* 2018;97(11):741–748.
2. Higdon ML, Higdon JA. Treatment of oncologic emergencies. *Am Fam Physician.* 2006;74(11):1873–1880.
3. Howard SC, Jones DP, Pui CH. The tumor lysis syndrome. *N Eng J Med.* 2011;364(19):1844–1854.

Severe Hypercalcemia of Malignancy

Presentation

Severe hypercalcemia of malignancy is a hypercalcemic crisis usually with serum Ca > 14 mg/dL and usually occurs in patients with breast cancer, lung cancer, and multiple myeloma, but can happen in any type of cancer.[1] Most commonly, it is due to parathyroid hormone–related protein in 80% of cases and less commonly due to bone invasion from osteolytic metastases in 20% of cases.[2]

Symptoms include generalized weakness, loss of appetite, nausea, vomiting, constipation, and decreased urinary output. Hypercalcemia of malignancy has poor prognosis.

Causes for Rapid Response Activation

Progressively worsening lethargy, confusion, bradycardia, heart block especially in elderly patients.

Actions

INITIAL MEASURES

1. Maintain continuous pulse oximetry.
2. Administer supplemental oxygen to maintain SpO_2 > 92%.
3. Maintain continuous cardiac monitoring.
4. Discontinue medications that could contribute to hypercalcemia, such as hydrochlorothiazide, calcium carbonate (antacid), vitamin A and D supplements, and lithium.

DIAGNOSTIC WORK-UP

1. Labs: BMP (elevated calcium), ionized calcium, phosphorus, PTH (parathyroid hormone), PTHrP (parathyroid hormone–related peptide), 1,25-dihydroxyvitamin D levels to screen for vitamin D–mediated hypercalcemia, which is typically seen in lymphomas.[3]
2. 12-Lead and rhythm EKG: shortening of QT interval, prolongation of PR interval, prolongation of QRS, ST changes, flat or inverted T-waves, and various degrees of AV block.

TREATMENT

1. Hydrate with 0.9% normal saline; avoid fluid overload.
2. Forced calciuresis can be achieved by using loop diuretic such as furosemide IV with IV fluid hydration in patients who experience fluid overload due to IV fluid hydration.[3]
3. Consult nephrologist for urgent dialysis if patient is unable to tolerate large volumes of fluids due to heart or renal failure.

4. Administer calcitonin 4–8 IU/kg SC or IM every 6–12 h as needed for hypocalcemic response; decrease in serum calcium occurs within 4 h of administration; it should not be administered > 48 h due to tachyphylaxis.[3]

5. Bisphosphonates will take 48–72 h before they reach full therapeutic effect:
   - Zoledronic acid 4 mg IV infusion over 15 min
   - Pamidronate 60–90 mg IV infusion over 2–4 h[3]

6. Administer denosumab (monoclonal antibody) 120 mg subcutaneously in patients refractory to bisphosphonates; effect will be seen within 2–4 days after administration.

References

1. Sohi R, Sheppard G. Hypercalcemia of malignancy: an emergency medicine simulation. *Cureus*. 2017;9(11), e1847.
2. Higdon ML, Atkinson CJ, Lawrence KV. Oncologic emergencies: recognition and initial management. *Am Fam Physician*. 2018;97(11):741–748.
3. Mirrakhimov A. Hypercalcemia of malignancy: an update on pathogenesis and management. *N Am J Med Sci*. 2015;7(11):483–493.

Syndrome of Inappropriate Antidiuretic Hormone (SIADH)

Presentation

SIADH in an oncologic patient is defined as an endocrine paraneoplastic syndrome of inappropriate production and release of antidiuretic hormone with resultant hyponatremia with serum sodium < 135 mEq/L, serum osmolality < 275 mOsm/kg, urine sodium > 40 mEq/L, and urine osmolality > 100 mOsm/kg.[1] It is most commonly associated with small cell lung cancer.[2] Other malignancies, such as head and neck tumors, extrapulmonary small cell cancers, and olfactory neuroblastomas, can also cause SIADH.[3]

Patient may present with gastrointestinal and neurological symptoms,[2] such as fatigue, nausea, vomiting, decreased appetite, muscle cramps, headache, and altered mental status.

Causes for Rapid Response Activation

Worsening altered mental status, such as confusion, delirium, obtundation and coma, seizure.

Actions

INITIAL MEASURES

1. Maintain continuous pulse oximetry.
2. Administer supplemental oxygen to maintain $SpO_2 > 92\%$.
3. Maintain continuous cardiac monitoring.
4. Consult nephrologist.

DIAGNOSTIC WORK-UP

Labs: BMP (hyponatremia), serum osmolality (low), urine sodium (high), urine osmolality (high).

TREATMENT

1. Correct serum sodium slowly: $< 10-12$ mEq/L/24 h and < 18 mEq/L/48 h, or $< 0.5-1$ mEq/L/h, to avoid central pontine myelinolysis; some authors recommend < 8 mEq/L/24 h.[4]
2. Monitor serum sodium very closely, every 2–4 h.
3. The goal of sodium correction is > 130 mEq/L.[3]
4. Oral water restriction 500 mL to 1 L a day is a first-line therapy in patients with mild-to-moderate symptoms.[2,4]

5. Use combination of low dose loop diuretic, for example, furosemide 20 mg IV one to two times daily and sodium chloride in the form of oral salt tablets or IV saline, if no improvement within 24–48 h of oral water restriction.[3,4]

6. In rare situations when patient has respiratory arrest, seizure, stupor, or coma due to acute hyponatremia (occurred within <24–48 h), consult nephrologist for 3% hypertonic saline administration:
   ▪ 3% hypertonic saline at 100 mL bolus is given in the first 3–4 h.[3]
   ▪ A rise of serum sodium by 3–4 mEq/L within the first few hours is reasonable[3]; however, total correction in the first 24 h still should not exceed 10–12 mEq.[4]
   ▪ Perform frequent sodium monitoring every 2 h.[3]
   ▪ The risk of treatment with 3% hypertonic saline is excessively rapid correction of serum sodium that can lead to central pontine myelinolysis.[4]

7. Consult nephrologist for consideration of vasopressin receptor antagonists approved by FDA in severe persistent SIADH such as:
   ▪ Conivaptan at loading dose of 20 mg IV over 30 min, followed by continuous infusion of 20 mg over 24 h, for no more than 4 days; in euvolemic and hypervolemic hyponatremia only.[4]
   ▪ Tolvaptan 15 mg PO once daily, titrating up to 60 mg PO daily; in euvolemic and hypervolemic patients only; avoid fluid restriction while establishing the maintenance dose.[4]
   ▪ The risk of treatment with vaptans is excessively rapid correction of serum sodium that can lead to central pontine myelinolysis.[4]
   ▪ Vaptans are nephrotoxic and hepatotoxic drugs and are not recommended in patients with creatinine clearance <30 mL/min, dialysis, or underlying liver disease.

References

1. Berardi R, Antonuzzo A, Blasi L, et al. Practical issues for the management of hyponatremia in oncology. *Endocrine*. 2018;61(1):158–164.
2. Higdon ML, Atkinson CJ, Lawrence KV. Oncologic emergencies: recognition and initial management. *Am Fam Physician*. 2018;97(11):741–748.
3. Yasir M, Mechanic OJ. *Syndrome of Inappropriate Antidiuretic Hormone Secretion*. StatPearls Publishing; 2020.
4. Thomas CP. *Syndrome of Inappropriate Antidiuretic Hormone Secretion*. Emedicine.medscape.com. Updated: August 16, 2019.

Febrile Neutropenia

Presentation

Febrile neutropenia is defined as a single axillary or oral temperature $\geq 101.3°F$ ($38.5°C$) or a sustained temperature $\geq 100.4°F$ ($38°C$) for 1 h, and an absolute neutrophil count (ANC) < 500 cells/mm^3 or an expected decrease of ANC to < 500 cells per mm^3 in the next 48 h, in a cancer patient on chemotherapy.[1] Neutropenia occurs due to bone marrow damage by cancer or chemotherapy and radiation. Damage to host barriers by chemotherapy and radiation leads to bacterial, fungal, and viral infections.

Febrile neutropenia can lead to severe sepsis and septic shock. Patients with significant comorbidities, renal insufficiency, hepatic insufficiency, and progressive cancer are at higher risk for having higher morbidity and mortality.

Causes for Rapid Response Activation

Hypotension.

Actions

INITIAL MEASURES

1. Maintain continuous pulse oximetry.
2. Administer supplemental oxygen to maintain $SpO_2 > 92\%$.
3. Maintain continuous cardiac monitoring.
4. Consult oncologist and infectious disease doctor early in the course of rapid response.

DIAGNOSTIC WORK-UP

1. Labs: CBC, CMP, lactic acid, procalcitonin, and urinalysis.
2. Blood cultures should be drawn, one from each lumen of a central line and one peripheral culture or two peripheral cultures if a central line is not present.[2]
3. Collect cultures from other sites, such as urine, stool (including *Clostridium difficile*), sputum, CSF, and wounds, as clinically indicated.
4. Order nasopharyngeal swab for COVID-19 and influenza as indicated in the setting of seasonal community-acquired respiratory illnesses.
5. Order chest X-ray.

TREATMENT

1. Empiric antibiotic treatment within 30 min of presentation will improve survival rate; the following antibiotics with antipseudomonal coverage are appropriate as monotherapy:
   - Piperacillin-tazobactam 4.5 g IV q 6 h
   - Cefepime 2 g IV q 8 h
   - Meropenem 1 g IV q 8 h
   - Imipenem-cilastatin 500 mg IV q 6 h[3]

2. Aminoglycoside can be added to any of the preceding antibiotics for dual therapy in patients with suspected or known multidrug resistance. Aminoglycoside options:
   - Gentamicin 2 mg/kg IV q 8 h or 5 mg/kg q 24 h
   - Amikacin 15 mg/kg/day IV divided q8–12 h
   - Tobramycin 2 mg/kg IV q 8 h[3]
3. Add vancomycin 15 mg/kg IV every 12 h:
   - Clinically suspected serious catheter-related infections (e.g., bacteremia, cellulitis)
   - Known colonization with penicillin- and cephalosporin-resistant pneumococci or methicillin-resistant *Staphylococcus aureus* (MRSA)
   - Blood culture positive for gram-positive bacteria
   - Hypotension
   - Severe mucositis, if prior fluoroquinolone prophylaxis provided[3]
4. In unstable patients with known history of prior infection or colonization with antibiotic-resistant organisms, modify initial antibiotic treatment:
   - MRSA (methicillin-resistant *Staphylococcus aureus*) or suspected catheter-related infection, skin or soft-tissue infection, pneumonia, or hemodynamic instability: vancomycin, linezolid, or daptomycin
   - VRE (vancomycin-resistant *Enterococcus*): linezolid or daptomycin
   - ESBL (extended-spectrum β-lactamase): carbapenem
   - KPC (Klebsiella *pneumoniae* carbapenemase): polymyxin-colistin or tigecycline[3]
5. Empiric antifungal treatment for patients with persistent fever for 4 days after initiation of antibacterial treatment:
   - *Candida*—fluconazole
   - *C. glabrata* or *C. krusei*—caspofungin
   - Aspergillus—voriconazole[4]
6. Administer filgrastim (granulocyte colony-stimulating factor) 5 μg/kg/day SC or IV no sooner than 24 h after chemotherapy completion, to shorten duration of neutropenia.[4]

References

1. Higdon ML, Atkinson CJ, Lawrence KV. Oncologic emergencies: recognition and initial management. *Am Fam Physician*. 2018;97(11):741–748.
2. Freifeld AG, Bow AJ, Sepkowitz KA, et al. Clinical practice guideline for the use of antimicrobial agents in neutropenic patients with cancer: 2010 update by the Infectious Diseases Society of America. *Clin Infect Dis*. 2011;52:e56–e93.
3. Denshaw-Burke M. *Neutropenic Fever Empiric Therapy*. Emedicine.medscape.com. Updated: November 16, 2019.
4. Lucas AJ, Olin JL, Coleman MD. Management and preventive measures for febrile neutropenia. *Pharm Therap*. 2018;43(4):228–232.

Acute Hyperviscosity Syndrome

Presentation

Acute hyperviscosity syndrome is characterized by elevated serum immunoglobulins that increase blood viscosity and decrease tissue perfusion. Waldenström macroglobulinemia is the most common cause of hyperviscosity syndrome.[1] Another cause is multiple myeloma. Hyperviscosity syndrome can also be caused by bone marrow hyperproliferative states such as leukemia, thrombocytosis, polycythemia, and myelodysplastic disorders.[1]

The classic triad of hyperviscosity includes mucosal bleeding, visual disturbances, and neurological abnormalities. Patients may present with epistaxis that is difficult to control, gingival bleeding, gastrointestinal bleeding, diplopia, blurry vision due to retinal hemorrhage, confusion, headache, lightheadedness, somnolence, or dyspnea due to heart failure or pulmonary hypertension.[2]

Causes for Rapid Response Activation

Bleeding (e.g., epistaxis that is difficult to control with direct pressure), worsening mental status, for example, somnolence progressing to stupor and coma, seizure, worsening hypoxia, dyspnea.

Actions

INITIAL MEASURES

1. Maintain continuous pulse oximetry.
2. Administer supplemental oxygen to maintain $SpO_2 > 92\%$.
3. Maintain continuous cardiac monitoring.
4. Consult oncologist early in the course of rapid response.

DIAGNOSTIC WORK-UP

1. Labs: CBC (hyperleukocytosis in leukemia, anemia), peripheral blood smear, CMP (hyperkalemia, hypercalcemia, total protein, albumin), phosphorus (hyperphosphatemia), coagulation studies (prothrombin time, activated partial thromboplastin time), immunoglobulin level (usually > 4000 mg/dL in hyperviscosity syndrome), viscosity (normal is 1.4–1.8 cP, patients become symptomatic with viscosity > 5 cP),[3] serum and urine electrophoresis for patients who have not been diagnosed with Waldenström macroglobulinemia or multiple myeloma.
2. Ophthalmoscopy: venous tortuosity, retinal hemorrhages, central retinal vein occlusion.[2]
3. Imaging: chest X-ray in patients with hypoxia and dyspnea, head CT scan or MRI in patients with neurological symptoms; contrast dye contraindicated in patients with multiple myeloma due to high risk for acute kidney injury.[3]

TREATMENT

1. Start plasmapheresis to reduce immunoglobulin level and subsequent plasma viscosity; do not wait for the results of the tests; one session that exchanges one volume of patient's plasma is required to stop mucosal hemorrhage; maximum of three sessions is required for viscosity level > 6 cP[4]; monitor for hypotension and allergic reactions.
2. In hyperleukocytosis due to leukemia with WBC > 100,000 cell/mL, processing ~1.5–2 total blood volumes for each leukapheresis to remove 30%–60% of the WBCs is recommended[3]; monitor for tumor lysis syndrome.
3. Withhold pRBC transfusion until WBC count is lowered; if unable to withhold transfusion, administer it by slow infusion.[3]
4. Start plateletpheresis for patients with thrombocytosis.
5. Start phlebotomy for polycythemia patients.

References

1. Higdon ML, Atkinson CJ, Lawrence KV. Oncologic emergencies: recognition and initial management. *Am Fam Physician*. 2018;97(11):741–748.
2. Gertz MA. Acute hyperviscosity: syndromes and management. *Blood*. 2018;132(13):1379–1385.
3. Hemingway TJ. *Hyperviscosity Syndrome*. Emedicine.medscape.com. Updated: December 11, 2019.
4. Ballestri M, Ferrari F, Magistroni R, et al. Plasma exchange in acute and chronic hyperviscosity syndrome: a rheological approach and guidelines study. *Ann Ist Super Sanita*. 2007;43(2):171–175.

Superior Vena Cava Syndrome

Presentation

In superior vena cava syndrome, the venous blood return to the heart is compromised by a mass compressing the superior vena cava in patients with cancer, for example, right upper lobe lung cancer or mediastinal lymphoma. Examples of nononcologic causes of superior vena cava syndrome include thrombosis from central venous instrumentation such as pacemaker or hemodialysis catheter.[1]

Symptoms include cough, hoarseness, dyspnea, orthopnea, stridor, chest pain, and facial, neck, and upper extremity edema. Laryngeal edema can lead to severe airway compromise. On examination, patient will have facial plethora and neck vein distention.[1]

Causes for Rapid Response Activation

Rarely this condition manifests as an emergency, but rapid response can be called for worsening facial edema, dyspnea, syncope, or symptoms of airway obstruction.

Actions

INITIAL MEASURES

1. Maintain continuous pulse oximetry.
2. Administer supplemental oxygen to maintain $SpO_2 > 92\%$.
3. Maintain continuous cardiac monitoring.
4. Elevate the head of the bed and have the patient sit upright to decrease venous pressure.
5. Consult oncologist, interventional radiologist, and cardiovascular surgeon early in the course of rapid response.

DIAGNOSTIC WORK-UP

1. Labs: CBC (leukopenia, anemia, thrombocytopenia), CMP (hypercalcemia), and coagulation studies (prothrombin time, activated partial thromboplastin time).
2. Chest X-ray may demonstrate lung mass, mediastinal widening, or pleural effusion.
3. Order ultrasound of jugular, subclavian, and axillary and innominate veins to detect thrombosis; is more appropriate for patients with mild symptoms.
4. Contrast-enhanced CT scan or MRI of chest will provide more information on the etiology, the location, and the extent of the venous obstruction and the presence of collaterals.[2]

TREATMENT

1. Start intubation and mechanical ventilation for patients with airway compromise; intubation may require anesthesiologist's assistance.
2. Administer diuretics such as furosemide 20–40 mg IV every 6–8 h until desired diuresis occurs, to decrease the volume of the fluid within the bloodstream; avoid hypovolemia.[2]

3. Administer steroids such as methylprednisolone 125 mg IV to reduce the swelling of the tumor; taper steroids slowly.[2]
4. Patient may need endovenous recanalization (mechanical thrombolysis, pharmacologic thrombolysis, balloon angioplasty) with SVC stent placement for rapid symptomatic relief.[3]
5. Thrombosis from central venous catheter is addressed with removal of the catheter along with anticoagulation therapy with heparin drip and catheter-directed thrombolysis with alteplase or thrombectomy.[4]
6. Patient may need radiation and chemotherapy to reduce malignant obstruction.[1]
7. Surgical bypass can be considered in patients who failed endovenous therapy.[5]

References

1. Higdon ML, Atkinson CJ, Lawrence KV. Oncologic emergencies: recognition and initial management. *Am Fam Physician*. 2018;97(11):741–748.
2. Drews RE, Rabkin DJ. *Malignancy-Related Superior Vena Cava Syndrome*. Uptodate.com. Updated: February 11, 2021.
3. Rizvi AZ, Kalra M, Bower TC, et al. Benign superior vena cava syndrome: stenting is now the first line of treatment. *J Vasc Surg*. 2008;47(2):372–380.
4. Kalra M, Sen I, Gloviczki P. Endovenous and operative treatment of superior vena cava syndrome. *Surg Clin North Am*. 2018;98(2):321–335.
5. Nickloes TA. *Superior Vena Cava Syndrome Treatment and Management*. Emedicine.medscape.com. Updated: March 27, 2020.

Malignant Epidural Spinal Cord Compression

Presentation

Malignant epidural spinal cord compression is most commonly caused by the extension of vertebral metastases or a fragment from a vertebral compression fracture into the spinal canal and can cause paralysis if untreated. It is most commonly associated with breast cancer. Multiple myeloma, lung cancer, lymphoma, renal cancer, and prostate cancer can also cause this oncologic emergency.[1]

Symptoms include progressive back pain, which can be localized or radicular, made worse with coughing, sneezing, straining, and lying down; bilateral extremity weakness; limb paresthesias; urinary retention; and urinary or fecal incontinence. On physical examination, there will be spinal tenderness to percussion of the involved vertebrae. Patients will have limited straight leg raising due to pain traveling down the asymptomatic limb. Patients will typically have hyperreflexia.[1]

Causes for Rapid Response Activation

Progressively worsening neurological changes.

Actions

INITIAL MEASURES

1. Maintain continuous pulse oximetry.
2. Administer supplemental oxygen to maintain $SpO_2 > 92\%$.
3. Maintain continuous cardiac monitoring.
4. Consult oncologist and neurosurgeon early in the course of rapid response.

DIAGNOSTIC WORK-UP

1. Plain spinal radiography may demonstrate osteolytic or osteoblastic lesions or vertebral collapse.
2. MRI of the spine is the imaging of choice.[2]
3. Order postvoid residual to assess urinary retention.

TREATMENT

1. Dexamethasone 4 mg IV q 4 h[3]
2. Radiation and/or chemotherapy
3. Surgical decompression

References

1. Higdon ML, Atkinson CJ, Lawrence KV. Oncologic emergencies: recognition and initial management. *Am Fam Physician.* 2018;97(11):741–748.
2. Borke J. *Spinal Cord Neoplasms.* Emedicine.medscape.com. Updated: July 17, 2019.
3. Kumar A, Weber MH, Gokaslan Z, et al. Metastatic spinal cord compression and steroid treatment: a systematic review. *Clin Spine Surg.* 2017;30(4):156–163.

Rapidly Accumulating Malignant Pericardial Effusion

Presentation

Malignant pericardial effusion occurs due to extension from an adjacent mediastinal mass or deposits from hematogenous or lymphatic metastatic spread that cause inflammation and obstruction of lymphatic drainage from the pericardial space. Rapid accumulation of fluid in the pericardial space will lead to both right and left ventricular failure due to decreased cardiac filling.[1]

Lung and breast cancers are the most common causes of malignant pericardial effusion. Other causes are cancers such as esophageal, Hodgkin and non-Hodgkin lymphomas, and leukemias and melanomas. This condition is associated with poor prognosis.[1]

Symptoms include dyspnea, pleuritic chest pain, cough, orthopnea, and peripheral edema. Severe cases will lead to shock. On physical examination, patients will have tachypnea; Beck's triad of tachycardia, hypotension, and muffled heart sounds; elevated JVP, and pulsus paradoxus.[1,2]

Causes for Rapid Response Activation

Progressively worsening dyspnea, chest pain, syncope.

Actions

INITIAL MEASURES

1. Maintain continuous pulse oximetry.
2. Administer supplemental oxygen to maintain $SpO_2 > 92\%$.
3. Maintain continuous cardiac monitoring.
4. Consult cardiovascular surgeon and oncologist emergently.

DIAGNOSTIC WORK-UP

1. 12-Lead EKG may be normal, or show sinus tachycardia, low QRS voltage, nonspecific ST- or T-wave changes, or electrical alternance.[2]
2. Chest X-ray will demonstrate widened mediastinum and pleural effusions.
3. Echocardiogram is the diagnostic modality of choice; echo will confirm pericardial effusion and will assess its size; the following signs are consistent with cardiac tamponade:
   - Collapse of the right atrium at end diastole and the right ventricle in early diastole
   - Reciprocal changes in left and right ventricular volumes with respiration
   - Increased respiratory variation of mitral and tricuspid valve inflow velocities
   - Inferior vena cava (IVC) dilatation with $< 50\%$ reduction in IVC diameter during inspiration[2,3]

TREATMENT

1. Administer IV fluids for hypovolemic patients with systolic blood pressure < 100 mmHg.[2]
2. Echo-guided pericardiocentesis will provide immediate relief of symptoms; indication for pericardiocentesis is symptomatic patient with evidence of chamber collapse on echo.[2]
3. Pigtail catheter may be placed into pericardial space for ongoing fluid removal until drainage is < 20–30 mL/24 h.[2]
4. Repeat echo after pericardiocentesis to:
   - Ensure adequate amount of pericardial fluid was removed
   - Monitor reaccumulation of pericardial fluid[2]
5. Submit pericardial fluid for Gram stain, bacterial and fungal cultures, and cytology; consider viral PCR if indicated.[2]
6. Pericardial sclerosis (with doxycycline or bleomycin) or surgical decompression therapies, such as pericardial "window," may be needed in patients expected to reaccumulate pericardial effusion.
7. Patient may need systemic chemotherapy and/or radiotherapy.

References

1. Higdon ML, Atkinson CJ, Lawrence KV. Oncologic emergencies: recognition and initial management. *Am Fam Physician.* 2018;97(11):741–748.
2. Petrofsky M. Management of malignant pericardial effusion. *J Adv Pract Oncol.* 2014;5(4):281–289.
3. Hoit BD. *Diagnosis and Treatment of Pericardial Effusion. UpToDate*; 2013. Uptodate.com.

CHAPTER 8

Infectious Disease Emergencies

Sepsis and Septic Shock

Presentation

Sepsis is a potentially fatal emergency leading to more than 200,000 deaths in the United States each year.[1] Following the convening of the Third International Consensus Definitions Task Force by the Society of Critical Care Medicine and the European Society of Intensive Care Medicine, the Surviving Sepsis Campaign published updated sepsis guidelines in 2016.[2]

According to 2016 guidelines, sepsis is defined as life-threatening organ dysfunction caused by a dysregulated host response to infection. Definitions such as Systemic Inflammatory Response Syndrome and Severe Sepsis were removed from the guidelines. The guidelines recommend to use the Sequential (Sepsis-Related) Organ Failure Assessment (SOFA) score to rapidly identify patients with sepsis. Septic shock is defined as sepsis with persistent hypotension requiring vasopressors to maintain mean arterial pressure (MAP) $\geq$ 65 mmHg and a serum lactate > 2 mmol/L (18 mg/dL) despite adequate volume resuscitation.[3]

Significant reduction in mortality was associated with early identification of sepsis, initiation of a 1-h care bundle, and rapid administration of broad-spectrum antibiotics. Risk factors for sepsis include ages 65–84,[1] chronic comorbidities, immunocompromised status, and traumatic injury.[2]

Symptoms include systemic symptoms such as fever, shaking chills, sweating, malaise, altered mental status, and localizing symptoms related to the source of infection. On examination, patient will have cold and clammy skin, tachycardia, tachypnea, and hypotension.

Causes for Rapid Response Activation

Tachycardia, hypotension, altered mental status.

Actions

INITIAL MEASURES

1. Maintain continuous pulse oximetry.
2. Administer supplemental oxygen to maintain SpO_2 > 92%.
3. Maintain continuous cardiac monitoring.
4. Perform quickSOFA (qSOFA) score for patients outside the ICU:
   - Elevated respiratory rate $\geq$ 22 breaths per minute
   - Altered mental status (Glasgow Coma Scale score < 15)
   - Systolic blood pressure of 100 mmHg or less
5. Calculate SOFA score for ICU patients based on the following factors:
   - PaO_2/FiO_2 (mmHg)
   - SaO_2/FiO_2

- Platelets × $10^3/mm^3$
- Bilirubin (mg/dL)
- Hypotension
- Glasgow Coma Scale
- Creatinine (mg/dL) or urine output (mL/day)

6. Patients with an increase of 2 or more in the SOFA score have an estimated in-hospital mortality of 10% due to sepsis and a 2- to 25-fold increased risk of death compared with patients with a SOFA score of < 2.[4]

DIAGNOSTIC WORK-UP

1. Labs: CBC (leukocytosis, left shift, bandemia, thrombocytopenia), CMP (hyperglycemia, organ dysfunction such as elevated creatinine or liver enzymes), procalcitonin (elevated in bacterial and fungal infection), lactate, coagulation studies (INR > 1.5), and UA (urinary tract infection).
2. Lactate levels greater than 2 mmol/L should be remeasured within 2–4 h to ensure the level is decreasing.
3. Order aerobic/anaerobic blood cultures prior to initiation of antibiotics, however, this should not delay administration of antibiotics within the first one hour of presentation.
4. Obtain other site-specific cultures, such as urine, sputum, and wound cultures.
5. Order EKG to assess for myocarditis or pericarditis.
6. Order site-specific imaging focused on source of infection.
7. Order site-specific invasive procedures to evaluate and/or treat source of infection—for example, transesophageal echo in patients with suspicion of valvular endocarditis; thoracentesis in patients with pleural effusion; paracentesis in patients with ascites, drainage of abscess, debridement and bone biopsy in osteomyelitis; and lumbar puncture.

TREATMENT

1. For fluid resuscitation, start normal saline 30 mL/kg IV within first 3 h for hypotension (mean arterial pressure ≤ 65 mmHg) or lactate ≥ 4 mmol/L.[5]
2. Further fluid administration is guided by:
   - Heart rate, blood pressure, arterial oxygen saturation, respiratory rate, temperature, and urine output
   - Passive leg raises
   - Bedside echocardiography
   - Other invasive and noninvasive techniques[5]
3. If hypotension (mean arterial pressure ≤ 65 mmHg) persists despite adequate volume resuscitation within first 3 h of presentation, add vasopressor and place arterial line.[5]
4. First-line vasopressors include:
   - Norepinephrine 5–15 μg/min IV infusion; usual maintenance dose range 2–80 μg/min[6]
   - Vasopressin 0.03 units/min to be added to decrease the dose of norepinephrine or to achieve the goal MAP ≥ 65 mmHg[5]
5. Second-line vasopressors include:
   - Epinephrine 1–15 μg/min IV infusion; usual maintenance dose range 1–40 μg/min[6]
6. Dobutamine is recommended for patients with persistent hypoperfusion despite adequate intravascular volume and vasopressor administration[5]:
   - Dobutamine 0.5–1 μg/kg/min IV infusion; usual maintenance dose range 2–20 μg/kg/min[6]
7. Initiate broad-spectrum empiric antimicrobials within 1 h of presentation[5]:
   - Administer piperacillin/tazobactam 4.5 g IV q 6 h[7] and vancomycin 15 mg/kg IV q 12 h with goal troughs of 15–20 mg/L.[8]
   - When candidemia is suspected, consider anidulafungin 200 mg IV day 1, followed by 100 mg IV daily starting day 2 thereafter.[9]

8. Deescalate antibiotics once pathogen and sensitivities are known.
9. Identify and control source of infection.
10. Remove old intravascular catheters.[5]
11. Administer hydrocortisone 200 mg IV daily in divided doses if fluid resuscitation and vasopressors fail to achieve hemodynamic stability, continue until vasopressors are no longer required.[1]
12. For blood products use:
    - Red blood cells if Hg <7 g/dL, except in active ischemic myocardial disease, acute hemorrhage, or persistent severe hypoxia.
    - FFP in patients with bleeding and coagulation abnormalities or planned procedures.
    - Platelet transfusion for levels $\leq 10{,}000/mm^3$ in the absence of bleeding or below $\leq 20{,}000/mm^3$ if there is a high risk of bleeding, and for patients with active bleeding or planned surgery/invasive procedures if platelets $\leq 50{,}000/mm^3$.
13. Start intubation and mechanical ventilation in sepsis-induced acute respiratory distress syndrome (ARDS):
    - Assist control or volume assist
    - Inspiratory to expiratory ratio (I/E) of 1:1 to 1:3
    - RR: 20–35 breaths per minute
    - Lower tidal volumes 6 mL/kg of predicted body weight:
        - Male: PBW (kg) = 50 + 2.3(height(in)-60)
        - Female: PBW (kg) = 45.5 + 2.3(height(in)-60)
    - Higher PEEP: start at 12 cm of H_2O, increase up to 28–30 cm of H_2O in severe ARDS
    - Plateau airway pressure $\leq 30\, cmH_2O$ to avoid barotrauma[10]
14. Assure prone positioning in patients with PaO_2/FIO_2 ratio ≤ 150 mmHg.[5]
15. Use conservative fluid infusion in patients with ARDS.[5]
16. Use neuromuscular blocking agents for ≤ 48 h in patients with sepsis-induced ARDS and PaO_2/FIO_2 ratio ≤ 150 mmHg.[5]
17. Glucose control:
    - Glucose levels should be checked every 1–2 h until a stable insulin regimen is reached and every 4 h thereafter.
    - Target blood glucose level is 110–180 mg/dL.[5]
18. Administer sodium bicarbonate in patients with pH <7.15.[5]

References

1. Epstein L, Dantes R, Magill S, Fiore A. Varying estimates of sepsis mortality using death certificates and administrative codes – United States, 1999–2014. *MMWR Morb Mortal Wkly Rep.* 2016;65:342–345.
2. Plevin R, Callcut R. Update in sepsis guidelines: what is really new? *Trauma Surg Acute Care Open.* 2017;2. https://doi.org/10.1136/tsaco-2017-000088, e000088.
3. Singer M, Deutschman CS, Seymour CW, et al. The third international consensus definitions for sepsis and septic shock (sepsis-3). *JAMA.* 2016;315:801–810.
4. Seymour CW, Liu VX, Iwashyna TJ, et al. Assessment of clinical criteria for sepsis: for the third international consensus definitions for sepsis and septic shock (sepsis-3). *JAMA.* 2016;315:762–774.
5. Rhodes A, Evans L, Alhazzani W, et al. Surviving Sepsis Campaign: international guidelines for management of sepsis and septic shock: 2016. *Crit Care Med.* 2017;45(3):486–552.
6. *Vasopressors and Inotropes in Treatment of Acute Hypotensive States and Shock: Adult Dose and Selected Characteristics.* Uptodate.com.
7. *Piperacillin-Tazobactam.* Reference.medscape.com.
8. *Vancomycin.* Reference.medscape.com.
9. *Anidulafungin.* Refence.medscape.com.
10. Saguil A, Fargo M. Acute respiratory distress syndrome: diagnosis and management. *Am Fam Physician.* 2020;101(12):730–738.

Acute Hypoxemic Respiratory Failure Due to Severe Pneumonia

Presentation

Community-acquired pneumonia (CAP) is one of the most common infectious diseases. The American Thoracic Society (ATS) and Infectious Diseases Society of America (IDSA) 2019 guidelines recommend to abandon the healthcare-associated pneumonia category and place emphasis on local epidemiology and validated risk factors to determine the need for MRSA or *P. aeruginosa* coverage.[1]

This section will cover severe CAP. According to ATS/IDSA 2019 guidelines, the definition of severe pneumonia includes either one major criterion or three or more minor criteria.

Minor criteria:

- Respiratory rate > 30 breaths/min
- PaO_2/FIO_2 ratio < 250
- Multilobar infiltrates
- Confusion/disorientation
- Uremia (blood urea nitrogen level > 20 mg/dL)
- Leukopenia (white blood cell count < 4000 cells/μL)
- Thrombocytopenia (platelet count < 100,000/μL)
- Hypothermia (core temperature < 36°C)
- Hypotension requiring aggressive fluid resuscitation

Major criteria:

- Septic shock with need for vasopressors
- Respiratory failure requiring mechanical ventilation[1]

Causes for Rapid Response Activation

Progressively worsening tachypnea, use of accessory respiratory muscles, cyanosis, tachycardia/bradycardia, hypotension, altered mental status.

Actions

INITIAL MEASURES

1. Maintain continuous pulse oximetry.
2. Administer supplemental oxygen to maintain SpO_2 > 90% or PaO_2 > 60–65 mmHg; transition to high flow oxygen when patient requires high flow rates.
3. Maintain continuous cardiac monitoring.
4. Position the patient to minimize aspiration risk.

DIAGNOSTIC WORK-UP

1. Labs: CBC with differential (leukocytosis, left shift, bandemia, thrombocytopenia), BMP, procalcitonin (elevated in bacterial/fungal infection), C-reactive protein (elevated), lactate, and ABG.

2. Obtain blood cultures, culture of respiratory secretions, and nasal MRSA PCR for the following patients:
    - With severe pneumonia, especially if intubated
    - Empirically treated for MRSA or *P. aeruginosa*
    - Previously infected with MRSA or *P. aeruginosa*
    - Who were hospitalized and received parenteral antibiotics within the last 90 days[1]
3. Order urine pneumococcal antigen in patients with severe pneumonia.[1]
4. Order urine *Legionella* antigen for:
    - Association with *Legionella* outbreak
    - Recent travel to an area with *Legionella* outbreak
    - Severe pneumonia[1]
5. Collect lower respiratory tract secretions for *Legionella* culture on selective media or *Legionella* nucleic acid amplification testing in patients with severe pneumonia.[1]
6. Order imaging:
    - Chest X-ray is the standard imaging test for establishing the diagnosis of pneumonia; viral pneumonia imaging will show bilateral, interstitial, symmetric, perihilar infiltrates; typical bacterial pneumonia will show focal segmental or lobar consolidation; atypical bacterial pneumonia will show focal segmental or bilateral interstitial infiltrates; *P. jiroveci* pneumonia will show bilateral patchy interstitial infiltrates.[2]
    - Chest ultrasonography may facilitate assessment for pneumonia at bedside.
    - Chest CT scan may be considered if chest X-ray is negative in immunocompromised patient.[2]

TREATMENT

1. Use heated/humidified oxygen via high flow nasal prongs.
2. Start suctioning to clear secretions.
3. Order chest physiotherapy.
4. Administer bronchodilators: albumin nebulizer 2.5–5 mg q 20 min for three doses; follow with 2.5–10 mg q 1–4 h PRN or 10–15 min by continuous nebulization.[3]
5. Administer *N*-acetylcysteine nebulizer:
    - 10% solution in 6–10 mL; administer 2–20 mL every 2–6 h
    - 20% solution in 3–5 mL; administer 1–10 mL every 2–6 h[4]
6. In severe pneumonia without risk factors for MRSA or *P. aeruginosa*, standard empiric therapy includes β-lactam/macrolide combination or β-lactam/respiratory fluoroquinolone.[1]
7. In severe pneumonia with risk factors for MRSA or *P. aeruginosa* (prior respiratory isolation of MRSA or *P. aeruginosa*, recent hospitalization and parenteral antibiotics, or locally validated risk factors are present), add coverage for MRSA and *P. aeruginosa*.[1]
8. Empiric antibiotic options for MRSA include:
    - Vancomycin 15 mg/kg IV every 12 h; adjust based on levels
    - Linezolid 600 mg PO/IV every 12 h[1]
9. Empiric antibiotic options for *P. aeruginosa* include:
    - Piperacillin-tazobactam 4.5 g IV every 6 h
    - Cefepime 2 g IV every 8 h
    - Ceftazidime 2 g IV every 8 h
    - Aztreonam 2 g IV every 8 h
    - Meropenem 500 mg IV every 8 h
    - Imipenem 500 mg IV every 6 h[1]
10. Deescalate antibiotics when pathogen and sensitivities are established.[1]
11. Consider corticosteroids in patients with refractory septic shock.[1]

12. Consult pulmonologist for consideration of bronchoscopy and therapeutic lavage.

13. Start intubation and mechanical ventilation for patients with hypoxia or hypercapnia refractory to noninvasive forms of oxygen delivery or inability to protect airway. Initial ventilator settings:
   - Mode of ventilation: assist control support.
   - Initial FiO_2: 100%; once patient stabilizes, titrate down to maintain SpO_2 at 92%–94%.
   - Tidal volume (VT) 6–8 mL/kg of predicted (ideal) body weight:
     - Male: PBW (kg) = 50 + 2.3(height(in)-60)
     - Female: PBW (kg) = 45.5 + 2.3(height(in)-60)
   - Maintain inspiratory plateau pressure ≤ 30 cmH$_2$O to avoid barotrauma.
   - RR: 12–16 breaths per minute.
   - Inspiratory to expiratory ratio (I/E) of 1:2.
   - PEEP: 5 cm of H$_2$O.[5]

References

1. Metlay JP, Waterer GW, Long AC, et al. Diagnosis and treatment of adults with community-acquired pneumonia. An official clinical practice guideline of the American Thoracic Society and Infectious Diseases Society of America. *Am J Respir Crit Care Med.* 2019;200(7):e45–e67.
2. Baer SL. *Community-Acquired Pneumonia.* Emedicine.medscape.com. Updated: October 31, 2019.
3. *Albuterol.* Reference.medscape.com.
4. *N-Acetylcysteine.* Reference.medscape.com.
5. Rammohan G, Meyers M. *Mechanical ventilation for pneumonia, acute respiratory distress syndrome and COVID-19.* Emergency Medicine Reports; 2020. Reliasmedia.com.

Hypovolemic Shock Due to Acute Infectious Diarrheal Illness

Presentation

Acute infectious diarrheal illness is common in adults. The most common etiology is viral gastroenteritis. Other etiology can be bacterial or parasitic. The most common bacterial causes of acute diarrhea in the United States are *Salmonella, Campylobacter, Shigella,* and Shiga toxin–producing *Escherichia coli* (STEC).[1] Elderly patients, patients residing in nursing homes, and recently hospitalized patients are at high risk for acute infectious diarrheal illness. Recent use of antibiotics and recent sick contacts are other risk factors.

Acute diarrheal illness is classified as noninflammatory and inflammatory syndromes. Noninflammatory syndrome is milder and is characterized by intestinal secretion without disruption in intestinal mucosa. Inflammatory syndrome is characterized by disruption of intestinal mucosa resulting in tissue invasion and tissue damage and generally leads to more severe disease.[2] Examples of pathogens causing noninflammatory syndrome include enterotoxigenic *E. coli, Bacillus cereus, Rotavirus, Norovirus,* and *Staphylococcus aureus.* Examples of pathogens causing inflammatory syndrome include STEC, *Salmonella, Shigella,* and *Clostridium difficile.* Symptoms of inflammatory diarrheal illness include fever, tenesmus, and grossly bloody stools.[2]

Patients with severe GI loss of fluids can develop hypovolemia with decreased tissue perfusion. Elderly patients are at higher risk. Symptoms of severe dehydration include thirst, dizziness, decreased urinary output, and altered mental status. On examination, these patients will have a generally ill appearance, dry mucous membranes, tachycardia, and hypotension.

Causes for Rapid Response Activation

Progressively worsening tachycardia, hypotension, altered mental status.

Actions

INITIAL MEASURES

1. Maintain continuous pulse oximetry.
2. Administer supplemental oxygen to maintain $SpO_2 > 90\%$ or $PaO_2 > 60–65$ mmHg; transition to high flow oxygen when patient requires high flow rates.
3. Maintain continuous cardiac monitoring.
4. Raise patient's legs to improve circulation.
5. Establish adequate IV access: two large-bore lines or central line.

DIAGNOSTIC WORK-UP

1. Labs: CBC with differential (leukocytosis/leukopenia, eosinophilia in parasitic infections, bandemia (especially due to *Shigella*), anemia, thrombocytopenia), CMP (electrolytes, renal function), procalcitonin (elevated in bacterial and fungal infection), and lactic acid.
2. Order fecal occult blood test.

3. Fecal lactoferrin (marker for leukocytes released by damaged intestinal mucosal cells) has higher specificity and sensitivity compared to fecal leukocytes.[2]

4. Polymerase chain reaction (PCR)–based multiple GI pathogen panels have improved turnaround time compared to stool cultures; however, "reflex stool cultures" are needed for taxonomic classification and susceptibility[3]; stool studies are recommended in the following situations:
   ■ Severe dehydration
   ■ Sepsis
   ■ Fever
   ■ Grossly bloody stool
   ■ Symptoms last > 3–7 days
   ■ Immunocompromised patients
   ■ Inflammatory diarrhea
   ■ Inflammatory bowel disease
   ■ Nosocomial diarrhea (onset after more than 3 days in the hospital, antibiotic use within 3 months)
   ■ Patients older than 65 years with significant comorbidities[4]

5. Order ova and parasites test in the following situations:
   ■ Diarrhea lasting > 7 days
   ■ Immunocompromised patients
   ■ Diarrhea associated with infants in daycare
   ■ Diarrhea associated with travel to mountainous regions
   ■ Diarrhea in patients with AIDS or men who have sex with men
   ■ Community waterborne outbreaks
   ■ Bloody diarrhea with few fecal leukocytes[5]

6. Patients with acquired immune deficiency syndrome (AIDS) with persistent diarrhea should undergo additional testing for organisms such as *Cryptosporidium*, *Cyclospora*, *Cystoisospora*, *Microsporidia*, *Mycobacterium avium* complex, and *Cytomegalovirus*.[6]

7. Test for *C. difficile* in symptomatic patients with new-onset ≥ 3 unformed stools in 24 h with:
   ■ History of diarrhea following antimicrobial use (within last 3 months)
   ■ Healthcare-associated diarrhea
   ■ Persistent diarrhea without an etiology and without recognized risk factors[6]

8. A single diarrheal stool specimen is recommended for detection of toxin or a toxigenic *C. difficile* strain (e.g., nucleic acid amplification testing); multiple specimens do not increase yield[6]; use rectal swab in patients with ileus.

9. Order blood cultures in febrile patients.

10. Imaging (ultrasonography, computed tomography, or magnetic resonance imaging) may detect small bowel/colonic wall circumferential thickening, intra-abdominal free air, and toxic megacolon.[6]

TREATMENT

1. Isotonic IV fluids such as normal saline or lactated Ringer's solution are recommended in severe dehydration, shock, ileus, or altered mental status; 1–2 L IV bolus is given initially, with close monitoring of vital signs, urinary output, and mental status.

2. Antimicrobial therapy for people with infections attributed to STEC O157 and other STEC that produce Shiga toxin 2 (or if the toxin genotype is unknown) should be avoided.[6]

3. Empiric antimicrobial therapy while waiting for the results of diagnostic work-up is recommended for the following patients with severe illness:
   ■ Immunocompromised patients
   ■ Ill immunocompetent patients with fever and bloody diarrhea[6]

4. Empiric antimicrobial therapy options should be provided depending on the local susceptibility patterns:
   - Ciprofloxacin 400 mg IV q 12 h
   - Azithromycin 500 mg IV daily[2]
5. Antimicrobial therapy should be narrowed when antimicrobial susceptibility testing results become available; more prolonged therapy might be required for immunocompromised patients:
   - *Campylobacter*:
     - Azithromycin 500 mg IV for 5 days
   - Non-Shiga *toxin*-producing *E. coli*:
     - Ciprofloxacin 400 mg IV q 12 h for 7 days
     - Azithromycin 500 mg IV daily for 5 days[2]
   - *Salmonella*:
     - Ciprofloxacin 400 mg IV q 12 h for 7 days
     - Azithromycin 500 mg IV daily for 5 days
     - Ceftriaxone 2 g IV daily for 7 days[2]
   - *Shigella*:
     - Ciprofloxacin 400 mg IV q 12 h for 7 days
     - Azithromycin 500 mg IV daily for 5 days[2]
   - *C. difficile*:
     - Discontinue all inciting antibiotics
     - Vancomycin 125 mg orally four times per day for 10–14 days[7]
   - First *recurrence* of CDI:
     - Oral vancomycin as a tapered and pulsed regimen: 125 mg po four times a day for 10–14 days, two times a day for a week, once per day for a week, and then every 2 or 3 days for 2–8 weeks
     - Fidaxomicin 200 mg twice daily for 10 days[7]
   - Multiple *recurrences* of CDI:
     - Fecal microbiota transplantation[7]
   - CDI ileus:
     - Vancomycin 500 mg orally four times per day and 500 mg in approximately 100 mL normal saline per rectum every 6 h as a retention enema and metronidazole 500 mg IV every 8 h
     - Consultation with general surgeon for severely ill patients for consideration of subtotal colectomy with preservation of the rectum[7]

References

1. Centers for Disease Control and Prevention. Preliminary FoodNet data on the incidence of infection with pathogens transmitted commonly through food—10 states, 2009. *MMWR Morb Mortal Wkly Rep.* 2010;59(14):418–422.
2. Barr W, Smith A. Acute diarrhea in adults. *Am Fam Physician.* 2014;89(3):180–189.
3. Dekker JP, Frank KM. Salmonella, Shigella and Yersinia. *Clin Lab Med.* 2015;35(2):225–246.
4. Bauer TM, Lalvani A, Fehrenbach J, et al. Derivation and validation of guidelines for stool cultures for enteropathogenic bacteria other than *Clostridium difficile* in hospitalized adults. *JAMA.* 2001;285(3):313–319.
5. Siegel DL, Edelstein PH, Nachamkin I. Inappropriate testing for diarrheal diseases in the hospital. *JAMA.* 1990;263(7):979–982.
6. Shane AL, Mody RK, Crump JA. 2017 Infectious Disease Society of America clinical practice guideline for the diagnosis and management of infectious diarrhea. *Clin Infect Dis.* 2017;65(12):e45–e80.
7. Aberra FN. What are IDSA/SHEA and the WSES diagnostic and treatment guidelines for Clostridium Difficile Infection (CDI)? Updated: July 25, 2019. Medscape.com..

Acute Respiratory Failure Due to Influenza Virus Infection

Presentation

Influenza is a common highly contagious airborne viral illness. It has seasonal activity and causes significant morbidity and mortality, especially in elderly patients and patients with chronic comorbidities. Three types of influenza viruses cause infection in humans: influenza A, B, and C. Influenza A infects multiple species, including humans, equines, swine, and birds. As Influenza A is more susceptible to antigenic variation, it contributes more to major pandemics.[1]

Common symptoms include chills related to fever, sweating, myalgias, malaise, sore throat, nasal discharge, cough, and headache. Some patients may have nausea, vomiting, and diarrhea. Symptoms usually continue for 2–8 days.[1] In severe pneumonia, patient will steadily deteriorate with development of dyspnea, tachypnea, and hypoxia. According to the 2010 guidelines of the World Health Organization (WHO),[2] severe influenza is defined as having at least one of the following clinical presentations:

- Dyspnea, tachypnea, or hypoxia
- Radiological signs of lower respiratory tract disease
- Central nervous system involvement (e.g., encephalopathy, encephalitis)
- Severe dehydration
- Acute renal failure
- Septic shock
- Exacerbation of underlying chronic disease, including asthma, chronic obstructive pulmonary disease (COPD), chronic hepatic or renal insufficiency, diabetes mellitus, or cardiovascular conditions
- Any other influenza-related condition or clinical presentation requiring hospital admission

Causes for Rapid Response Activation

Progressively worsening tachypnea, dyspnea, hypoxia, altered mental status.

Actions

INITIAL MEASURES

1. Maintain continuous pulse oximetry.
2. Administer supplemental oxygen to maintain $SpO_2 > 90\%$ or $PaO_2 > 60–65\,mmHg$; transition to high flow oxygen when patient requires high flow rates.
3. Maintain continuous cardiac monitoring.

DIAGNOSTIC WORK-UP

1. Order influenza A and B tests: reverse transcription-polymerase chain reaction (RT-PCR) or viral culture of nasopharyngeal or throat secretions; rapid diagnostic tests for influenza usually have a 30-min turnaround time.[3]
2. Obtain sputum and blood cultures in superimposed bacterial pneumonia.
3. Order nasal MRSA PCR.
4. Check for urine streptococcal and *Legionella* antigens (see the earlier section on severe pneumonia for indications).
5. Labs: CBC (leukopenia, thrombocytopenia, leukocytosis in superimposed bacterial infection), CMP (electrolyte abnormalities, renal failure), and procalcitonin (elevated in superimposed bacterial or fungal infection).
6. Order chest X-ray: clear lungs or minimal bilateral symmetrical interstitial infiltrates in early disease; bilateral patchy infiltrates later in the course of illness; in superimposed bacterial pneumonia, chest X-ray will demonstrate nonsegmental homogeneous consolidation involving one, or less commonly, multiple lobes.[3]
7. CT scan of chest will show multifocal ground glass opacities; lobar consolidation will suggest superimposed bacterial pneumonia.

Treatment

1. As patients with severe influenza are at high risk of developing acute respiratory distress syndrome (ARDS), use IV fluids cautiously.
2. Start antiviral treatment as soon as possible (most effective if started within 48 h of symptom onset) for hospitalized patients regardless of illness duration:
   - Oseltamivir 75 mg orally twice daily for 5 days; adjust dose to renal function
   - Peramivir 600 mg IV single dose (for patients who are unable to take oseltamivir orally); adjust dose to renal function
   - Zanamivir 10 mg inhalation twice daily for 5 days (contraindicated in intubated patients, not recommended in patients with asthma or COPD)[4]
3. If clinical course remains severe, duration of the antiviral treatment can be extended until clinical improvement.[2]
4. Investigate and empirically treat bacterial co-infection, for example, bacterial pneumonia in the following patients:
   - Patients presenting initially with severe influenza (extensive pneumonia, respiratory failure, hypotension, fever)
   - Patients who deteriorate after initial improvement, particularly those treated with antivirals
   - Patients who fail to improve after 3–5 days of antiviral treatment[4]
5. Commonly isolated bacteria in patients with influenza complicated by bacterial pneumonia are *Staphylococcus aureus* (including MRSA), *Streptococcus pneumonia*, *Streptococcus pyogenes*, and *Moraxella catarrhalis*,[2] empiric antibiotic options for which (except MRSA) include:
   - Ampicillin/sulbactam 3 g IV q 6 h for 7 days
   - Ceftriaxone 2 g IV daily for 7 days
   - Levofloxacin 750 mg IV daily for 5 days
6. Patients with suspected MRSA pneumonia should preferably be treated with linezolid due to superiority in treatment for MRSA pneumonia and decreased risk for nephrotoxicity[5]:
   - Linezolid 600 mg PO/IV q 12 h for 10 days
   - In case of contraindications for linezolid: vancomycin 15 mg/kg IV every 12 h; dose adjusted based on trough levels

7. Avoid corticosteroids unless there are other indications for them, such as asthma, COPD, or adrenal insufficiency.[2,4]

8. High-flow nasal cannula is preferred noninvasive respiratory support in patients with Influenza.[5]

9. Consider BiPAP in patients with asthma or COPD exacerbation[5]; however, if patient has evidence of ARDS, invasive PPV is the only strategy that improves mortality.

10. Start intubation and mechanical ventilation for patients with progressive hypoxia/hypercapnia despite optimal use of noninvasive respiratory support; ventilatory management principles for ARDS can be adopted in severe influenza.[6]

11. Initial ventilator settings:
    - Mode of ventilation: volume assist control.
    - Initial FiO_2: 100%; once the patient stabilizes, titrate it down to maintain SpO_2 at 88%–95% or PaO_2 55–80 mmHg.
    - PEEP: 18–24 cm of H_2O; titrate down as you titrate down FiO_2.
    - Tidal volume (VT) 6 mL/kg of predicted (ideal) body weight:
        - Male: PBW (kg) = 50 + 2.3(height(in)-60)
        - Female: PBW (kg) = 45.5 + 2.3(height(in)-60)
    - RR: 14–22 breaths per minute.
    - Inspiratory to expiratory ratio (I/E) of 1:2.
    - Maintain plateau pressure (Pplat) ≤ 30 cmH$_2$O to avoid barotrauma.
    - Monitor clinical response, Pplat, and ABGs closely.[7]

References

1. Gaitonde DY, Moore FC, Morgan MK. Influenza: diagnosis and treatment. *Am Fam Physician.* 2019;100(12):751–758.

2. Choi WS, Baek JH, Seo YB, et al. Severe influenza treatment guideline. *Korean J Intern Med.* 2014;29(1):132–147.

3. Nguyen HH. Influenza. Emedicine.medscape.com Updated: August 7, 2020..

4. Uyeki T, Bernstein HH, Bradley JS, et al. Clinical practice guidelines by Infectious Diseases Society of America: 2018 update on diagnosis, treatment, chemoprophylaxis and institutional outbreak management of seasonal influenza. *Clin Infect Dis.* 2019;68(6):e1–e47.

5. Farkas J. *Severe Influenza. Internet Book of Critical Care (IBCC)*; 2019. Emcrit.org.

6. Phua GC, Govert J. Mechanical ventilation in an airborne epidemic. *Clin Chest Med.* 2008;29(2):323–328.

7. Siegel MD, Hyzy RC. Ventilator management strategies for adults with acute respiratory distress syndrome. Uptodate.com. Last updated: November 26, 2019..

Acute Respiratory Failure Due to COVID-19 (Coronavirus Disease of 2019) Pneumonia

Presentation

Severe acute respiratory syndrome coronavirus 2 (SARS-CoV-2) is a highly contagious respiratory disease that can spread in aerosols. Mean incubation period is 5 days; however, it can range from 2 days to 2 weeks.[1] The disease ranges from asymptomatic to severe illness with acute respiratory failure, multiorgan failure, and death. Initial symptoms may include fever, chills, sore throat, nasal congestion, cough, shortness of breath, loss of taste and smell, headache, nausea, vomiting, and diarrhea. Severe cases are mostly reported in patients older than 55 years with significant comorbidities, including obesity.[1]

In this chapter we will only address management of severe (RR > 30 breaths/min, severe respiratory distress or SpO_2 < 90%) and critical (presence of ARDS, respiratory failure requiring ventilation, sepsis or septic shock) COVID-19.

Causes for Rapid Response Activation

Rapidly worsening dyspnea, tachypnea, hypoxia.

Actions

INITIAL MEASURES

1. Maintain continuous pulse oximetry.
2. Administer supplemental oxygen to maintain SpO_2 > 92%–96% or PaO_2 > 60–65 mmHg; transition to high flow oxygen when patient requires high flow rates.
3. Maintain continuous cardiac monitoring.

DIAGNOSTIC WORK-UP

1. Order SARS-CoV-2 test (viral nucleic acid or antigen detection test).[1]
2. Other labs include CBC (leukopenia, lymphopenia); CMP (elevated LFTs); coagulation studies (PT, aPTT); inflammatory markers such as CRP, LDH, ferritin, D-dimer, fibrinogen, and IL-6 (if elevated, associated with increased risk of ARDS and death)[2,3]; ABG; and BNP (BNP < 100 pg/mL in a patient with hypoxia and bilateral pulmonary infiltrates supports ARDS rather than cardiogenic pulmonary edema).[4]
3. Order chest X-ray: bilateral consolidation and diffuse ground-glass opacities with highest severity around days 10–12 following the onset of symptoms.[1]
4. Consider chest CT scan: ground-glass and fine reticular opacities with mostly peripheral distribution and vascular thickening.[1]
5. Order compression Doppler ultrasound (US) of extremities when DVT is suspected.
6. Order chest CTA in patients with elevated D-dimer to rule out pulmonary embolism.

TREATMENT

1. Prone positioning for awake spontaneously breathing patient is associated with improved oxygenation and a lower rate of intubation,[5] however, overall evidence is insufficient, awaiting the results of ongoing RCT's.

2. High flow nasal cannula will deliver heated humidified oxygen through large-bore nasal prongs; oxygen flow rate can be titrated up to 50–60 L/min to maintain SpO_2 of 88%–95%; this mode is associated with improved patient comfort as it allows patient to talk, eat, and move around.[4]

3. As patients with severe COVID-19 pneumonia are at high risk for ARDS, a fluid-conservative strategy is preferred (improved oxygenation index, lower lung injury score, and increase in ventilator-free days); closely monitor urine output; consider diuretic to maintain low normal fluid balance.[6]

4. Administer dexamethasone 6 mg PO/IV daily for 10 days or until discharge (or equivalent glucocorticoid if dexamethasone is not available) for all patients with RR > 30 breaths/min, severe respiratory distress or SpO_2 < 90% on room air.[7]

5. Equivalent glucocorticoids if dexamethasone is not available include:
   - Methylprednisolone 32 mg PO/IV daily
   - Prednisone 40 mg PO daily[7]

6. Remdesivir (antiviral agent) is recommended for patients with severe COVID-19 (RR > 30 breaths/min, severe respiratory distress or SpO_2 < 90% on room air) and should ideally be started within 72 h of positive COVID-19 test, it is no longer recommended in adults undergoing mechanical ventilation.[7]

7. Convalescent plasma is recommended by IDSA only in the context of a clinical trial.[7]

8. BiPAP/CPAP is administered by full facemask for patients with progressive hypoxia despite optimal use of high flow oxygen.

9. Start intubation and mechanical ventilation for patients with progressive hypoxia/hypercapnia despite optimal use of noninvasive respiratory support.

10. Initial ventilator settings:
    - Mode of ventilation: volume assist control.
    - Initial FiO_2: 100%; once patient stabilizes, titrate it down to maintain SpO_2 at 88%–95% or PaO_2 55–80 mmHg.
    - PEEP: 18–24 cm of H_2O; titrate down as you titrate down FiO_2.
    - Tidal volume (VT) 6 mL/kg of predicted (ideal) body weight:
      - Male: PBW (kg) = 50 + 2.3(height(in)-60)
      - Female: PBW (kg) = 45.5 + 2.3(height(in)-60)
    - RR: 14–22 breaths per minute.
    - Inspiratory to expiratory ratio (I/E) of 1:2.
    - Maintain plateau pressure (Pplat) ≤ 30 cmH₂O to avoid barotrauma.
    - Monitor clinical response, Pplat, and ABGs closely.[8]
    - Prone ventilation for 12–16 h/day is suggested.

11. Administer prophylactic dose anticoagulation with enoxaparin, fondaparinux, or heparin (if CrCl < 30 mL/min) for patients with severe and critical COVID-19, in the absence of contraindications.[7]

12. Administer therapeutic dose of anticoagulation for patients with documented or presumptive pulmonary embolism or deep vein thrombosis.

References

1. Cennimo DJ. *Coronavirus Disease 2019 (COVID-19)*. Emedicine.medscape.com. Updated: December 19, 2020.
2. Asghar MS, Haider Kazmi SJ, Khan N, et al. Poor prognostic biochemical markers predicting fatalities caused by COVID-19: a retrospective observational study from a developing country. *Cureus*. 2020;12(8), e9575.

3. Mughal M, Kaur IP, Jaffery A, et al. Can inflammatory markers predict the successful extubation in patients with COVID-19? *Chest.* 2020;158(4):A600.

4. Harman EM. *Acute Respiratory Distress Syndrome (ARDS).* Emedicine.medscape.com. Updated: March 27, 2020.

5. Thompson AE, Ranard BL, Wei Y, et al. Prone positioning in awake, nonintubated patients with COVID-19 hypoxemic respiratory failure. *JAMA Intern Med.* 2020;180(11):1537–1539.

6. Wiedemann HP, Wheeler AP, Bernard GR, et al. Comparison of two fluid-management strategies in acute lung injury. *N Engl J Med.* 2006;354(24):2564–2575.

7. Alhazzani W, Evans L, Alshamsi F, et al. Surviving sepsis campaign guidelines on the management of adults with coronavirus disease 2019 (COVID-19) in the ICU: first update. *Crit Care Med.* 2021;49(3):e219–e234.

8. Siegel MD, Hyzy RC. *Ventilator Management Strategies for Adults With Acute Respiratory Distress Syndrome.* Uptodate.com. Last updated: November 26, 2019.

CHAPTER 9

Management of Postprocedural Complications in Hospitalized Patients

Tracheostomy Basics

The most common indications for tracheostomy:

1. Need for comfortable airway for prolonged mechanical ventilation in patients who have difficulty weaning off a ventilator; tracheostomy allows patients to perform daily activities; American College of Chest Physicians recommends tracheostomy placement in patients who will require mechanical ventilation for more than 7–14 days.
2. Bypass glottic or supraglottic pathologic conditions such as stenosis from prolonged intubation, neoplasm (e.g., laryngeal carcinoma), and bilateral vocal cord paralysis.
3. Access for pulmonary toilet to remove tracheal secretions and protection from aspiration in patients with chronic dysphagia and inability to handle secretions.
4. Failure to protect the airway, such as upper airway foreign body that cannot be dislodged with Heimlich maneuver; comminuted facial fractures; severe trauma to tongue, mandible, thyroid, or cricoid cartilages; or burns.
5. Advanced neuromuscular disorders such as multiple sclerosis.
6. Severe sleep apnea refractory to CPAP (continuous positive airway pressure) machine treatment.

The trachea is D-shaped in cross-section and is 11 cm in length. Tracheostomies are placed surgically or percutaneously. The end of the tracheostomy tube should be 2–3 cm from the carina, which will prevent the tube from entering the mainstem bronchus with neck flexion. In patients with average body habitus, usually a size 6 Shiley tube is used for women and a size 8 Shiley tube is used for men. It normally takes 7–10 days for the track to mature. After the tracheostomy tube is removed (decannulation), the hole closes within a week.

There are cuffed and uncuffed tracheostomy tubes. Patients with newly formed tracheostomy dependent on positive-pressure ventilation and with high risk of aspiration will require cuffed tracheostomy tubes. Even when deflated, cuffs can irritate tracheal mucosa, worsen tracheal secretions, and sometimes cause pressure ischemia and necrosis or even erosion into nearby vessels.

A flange is used to secure the tracheostomy tube with ties and prevents the tube from descending into the trachea. The information on the type and size of the tube is imprinted on the surface of the flange. The outer cannula is the main part of the tracheostomy tube. The inner cannula is removable. Removing the inner cannula allows clearing of secretions to prevent mucus plugging. Some inner tubes are fenestrated. Fenestrated tubes allow effective cough and speech. Fenestrated tubes are contraindicated in patients dependent on positive-pressure ventilation. Pilot balloons are attached to cuffed tubes. An obturator is placed inside the outer cannula during the insertion of the tube into the trachea. The adaptor is a 15-mm hub that is connected to the tracheostomy tube to allow attachment to the ventilator when patient is in acute respiratory failure.

Further Reading

Lindman JP, Soo Hoo GW. *Tracheostomy.* Emedicine.medscape.com. Updated: December 28, 2018.

Short-Term Tracheostomy Complication (< 7 Days): Accidental Decannulation (Removal) of the Tracheostomy Tube

Presentation

Tube decannulation is common. Causes for decannulation include loose tracheostomy tube ties especially in the setting of forceful coughing. Conditions that could contribute to tube decannulation include obesity, neck edema, altered mental status, and increased pulmonary secretions.

Causes for Rapid Response Activation

Tracheostomy-dependent patient will develop symptoms like dyspnea, stridor, cyanosis, and hypoxia.

Actions

1. Look for the chest to rise, listen for breath sounds from the tracheostomy tube, and using your hand, feel for air coming from nose, mouth, or tracheostomy tube.
2. Maintain continuous pulse oximetry.
3. Maintain continuous cardiac monitoring.
4. Use end tidal CO_2 waveform capnography when available; exhaled carbon dioxide indicates patent or partially patent airway.
5. Apply high flow oxygen both to face and tracheostomy site to maintain $SpO_2 > 92\%$ or $PaO_2 > 60\,mmHg$.
6. Do not attempt to reinsert the tracheostomy tube into the tract to avoid inadvertent placement of the tube into the anterior mediastinal space, bypassing the airway.
7. Replacement of a decannulated tracheostomy tube < 7 days should be attempted only under direct visualization; therefore, obtain STAT ENT/anesthesia consult.
8. In the meantime, proceed with oral intubation to secure the airway for tracheostomy-dependent patients.

Further Reading

1. *National Tracheostomy Safety Project.* www.tracheostomy.org.uk.
2. McGrath B, Bates L, Atkinson D, Moore J. Multidisciplinary guidelines for the management of tracheostomy and laryngectomy airway emergencies. *Anaesthesia.* 2012;67(9):1025–1041.
3. O'Connor HH, White AC. Tracheostomy decannulation. *Respir Care.* 2010;55(8):1076–1081.

Short-Term Tracheostomy Complication (< 7 Days): Tracheostomy Site Hemorrhage

Presentation

Incidence is approximately 5% of tracheostomies performed in adult ICU.[1] Most common causes include manipulation of the tracheostomy tube and suctioning and could also be triggered by coughing and hypertension. Additional factors contributing to hemorrhage are tracheitis, granulation tissue, infection of the stoma, bleeding thyroid vessels, or ulcer from an ill-fitting tube. Symptoms include bleeding at the site of the stoma, bleeding from the lumen of the tracheostomy tube, oozing from the surgical site, nasopharyngeal and/or oropharyngeal bleeding, or aspiration of blood.

Causes for Rapid Response Activation

All cases of tracheostomy site hemorrhage must be considered a sentinel bleed and merit a rapid response call. The source of bleeding must be identified by exploration of the tracheostomy site, even if bleeding resolves.

Actions

1. Wear protective equipment such as gloves, gown, and face shield or goggles.
2. Maintain continuous pulse oximetry.
3. Maintain continuous cardiac monitoring.
4. Use end tidal CO_2 waveform capnography when available; exhaled carbon dioxide indicates patent or partially patent airway.
5. Apply high flow oxygen to both face and tracheostomy site to maintain $SpO_2 > 92\%$ or $PaO_2 > 60$ mmHg.
6. Look for the chest to rise, listen for breath sounds from the tracheostomy tube, and using your hand, feel for air coming from nose, mouth, or tracheostomy tube.
7. Suction blood clots.
8. Apply direct pressure with or without hemostatic dressing; you can use antibiotic-impregnated gauze (Iodophor) for local packing.
9. Cauterize the bleeding vessels with silver nitrate.
10. Administer anti-staphylococcal antibiotic while the packing is in place:
    - Cefazolin 2 g IV q 8 h[2]
    - Nafcillin 1 g IV q 4 h[3]
11. STAT CBC, coagulation studies, and type and cross.
12. Hold and reverse anticoagulation and correct underlying coagulopathy.
13. STAT ENT/anesthesia/vascular surgeon consult.

14. Transport the patient to operating room for exploration of the tracheostomy site with a fiberoptic bronchoscope to identify sources such as infection, granulation tissue, and tumor invasion; angiography may be needed to identify the source of bleeding, followed by the definitive repair, for example, ligation of thyroid artery if the source of bleeding is thyroid artery.

References

1. Bradley PJ. Bleeding around a tracheostomy wound: what to consider and what to do? *J Lanryngol Otol.* 2009;123(9):952–956.
2. *Cefazolin.* www.antimicrobe.org.
3. *Nafcillin.* www.antimicrobe.org.

Long-Term Tracheostomy Complication (> 7 Days): Blockage of the Tracheostomy Tube

Presentation

Common cause of respiratory compromise. Causes include mucus plug, thick secretions, and blood clots.

Causes for Rapid Response Activation

Shortness of breath, increased work of breathing, abnormal breath sounds, tachypnea, tachycardia, hypoxia. Late signs include cyanosis, bradycardia, and apnea.

Actions

1. Maintain continuous pulse oximetry.
2. Maintain continuous cardiac monitoring.
3. Use end tidal CO_2 waveform capnography when available; exhaled carbon dioxide indicates patent or partially patent airway.
4. Apply high flow oxygen to both face and tracheostomy site to maintain $SpO_2 > 92\%$ or $PaO_2 > 60\,mmHg$.
5. Look for the chest to rise, listen for breath sounds from the tracheostomy tube, and using your hand, feel for air coming from nose, mouth, or tracheostomy tube.
6. Obtain immediate access to tracheostomy equipment kit.
7. Remove inner cannula, speaking valve/cap, and humidifying device if present.
8. Pass a suction catheter to perform tracheal suction.
9. If you are unable to pass the catheter due to obstruction, deflate the cuff to allow extra room for patient to ventilate unaided.
10. If patient is not improving, remove and replace the tracheostomy tube with a smaller diameter tracheostomy tube using a bougie or fiberoptic scope.
11. If patient is unable to ventilate (not breathing) after re-cannulation of the tracheostomy tube or failed attempted re-cannulation, use primary emergency oxygenation maneuvers, such as:
    - Oral airway maneuvers, such as BVM (bag-valve-mask) or LMA (laryngeal mask airway) while covering stoma with a gauze and tape or with a hand to prevent air leak
    - Stoma ventilation such as pediatric facemask or LMA (laryngeal mask airway) to stoma
12. If that fails, attempt secondary emergency oxygenation maneuvers, such as:
    - Oral intubation with a long uncut tube to advance 2 cm beyond the stoma
    - Intubation of the stoma with small tracheostomy tube (5.5/6.0 cuffed tracheal tube) using a bougie or fiberoptic scope; obtain chest X-ray for confirmation

Further Reading

1. *National Tracheostomy Safety Project.* www.tracheostomy.org.uk.
2. McGrath B, Bates L, Atkinson D, Moore J. Multidisciplinary guidelines for the management of tracheostomy and laryngectomy airway emergencies. *Anaesthesia.* 2012;67(9):1025–1041.

Long-Term Tracheostomy Complication (> 7 Days): Accidental Decannulation (Removal) of the Tracheostomy Tube

Presentation

Tube decannulation is common. Causes for decannulation include loose tracheostomy tube ties especially in the setting of forceful coughing. Conditions that could contribute to tube decannulation include obesity, neck edema, altered mental status, and increased pulmonary secretions.

Causes for Rapid Response Activation

Tracheostomy-dependent patient will develop symptoms like dyspnea, stridor, cyanosis, and hypoxia.

Actions

1. Maintain continuous pulse oximetry.
2. Maintain continuous cardiac monitoring.
3. Use end tidal CO_2 waveform capnography when available; exhaled carbon dioxide indicates patent or partially patent airway.
4. Apply high flow oxygen both to face and tracheostomy site to maintain $SpO_2 > 92\%$ or $PaO_2 > 60\,mmHg$.
5. Look for the chest to rise, listen for breath sounds from the tracheostomy tube, and using your hand, feel for air coming from nose, mouth, or tracheostomy tube.
6. Obtain immediate access to a tracheostomy kit.
7. With the obturator in place, insert the tracheostomy tube of the same size gently but firmly into the patient's airway, remove the obturator, and inflate the cuff if present.
8. If the tube of the same size does not fit into the stoma, attempt to insert the next size down.
9. If failed, place a bougie into the tract to ensure the tract remains open.
10. Place a tracheostomy tube over the bougie using a Seldinger technique, with the tube pointed perpendicular to the stoma.
11. Once the tracheostomy tube is in place, the bougie can be removed.
12. Check tube position by auscultating the chest to ensure patent airway.
13. Once the tracheostomy tube is inserted, replace the oxygen via the tracheostomy tube or reattach the ventilator.

14. If attempted replacement failed, use primary emergency oxygenation maneuvers, such as:
  - Oral airway maneuvers, such as BVM (bag-valve-mask) or LMA (laryngeal mask airway) while covering stoma with a hand
  - Stoma ventilation such as pediatric facemask or LMA (laryngeal mask airway) to stoma

15. If that fails, attempt secondary emergency oxygenation maneuvers, such as:
  - Oral intubation with a long uncut tube to advance 2 cm beyond the stoma
  - Intubate the stoma with small tracheostomy tube (5.5/6.0 cuffed tracheal tube) using a bougie or fiberoptic scope; obtain chest X-ray for confirmation

Further Reading

1. *National Tracheostomy Safety Project.* www.tracheostomy.org.uk.
2. McGrath B, Bates L, Atkinson D, Moore J. Multidisciplinary guidelines for the management of tracheostomy and laryngectomy airway emergencies. *Anaesthesia.* 2012;67(9):1025–1041.
3. O'Connor HH, White AC. Tracheostomy decannulation. *Respir Care.* 2010;55(8):1076–1081.

Long-Term Tracheostomy Complication (> 7 Days): Tracheo-Esophageal Fistula

Presentation

This complication is rare with an incidence < 1%.[1] It occurs as a result of an injury to the tracheal wall from the tracheostomy tube or high cuff pressure during tube movements caused by frequent dressing changes or suctioning. Symptoms may include cough, chocking, shortness of breath with oral intake, and recurrent aspiration pneumonia. Patients with poorly controlled diabetes, poor nutrition, anemia, or steroid therapy may have higher risk for this complication.[2]

Causes for Rapid Response Activation

Progressively worsening dyspnea and hypoxia.

Actions

1. Maintain continuous pulse oximetry.
2. Maintain continuous cardiac monitoring.
3. Use end tidal CO_2 waveform capnography when available; exhaled carbon dioxide indicates patent or partially patent airway.
4. Apply high flow oxygen to both face and tracheostomy site to maintain SpO_2 > 92% or PaO_2 > 60 mmHg.
5. Look for the chest to rise, listen for breath sounds from the tracheostomy tube, and using your hand, feel for air coming from nose, mouth, or tracheostomy tube.
6. A barium swallow study with a water-soluble contrast can confirm the presence of tracheo-esophageal fistula.
7. Small defects may heal spontaneously.
8. Consult pulmonologist or anesthesiologist for fiberoptic bronchoscopy, which may demonstrate air bubbles at the site of the fistula and a defect over the posterior wall of the trachea.
9. Initially, patient will need insertion of a new tracheostomy tube with the cuff positioned below the fistula, and nutrition will be provided through percutaneous feeding gastrostomy or a jejunostomy tube.
10. Patients who are unable to tolerate tracheal reconstruction surgery may be treated with double esophageal and endotracheal self-expandable metallic stents.
11. Definitive treatment includes tracheal resection with anastomosis and primary esophageal closure performed in a staged manner.[3]

References

1. Epstein SK. Late complications of tracheostomy. *Respir Care.* 2005;50(4):542–549.
2. Sanwal MK, Ganjoo P, Tandon MS. Posttracheostomy tracheoesophageal fistula. *J Anaesthesiol Clin Pharmacol.* 2012;28(1):140–141.
3. Chua AP, Dalal B, Mehta AC. Tracheostomy tube induced tracheoesophageal fistula. *J Bronchology Interv Pulmonol.* 2009;16(3):191–192.

Long-Term Tracheostomy Complication (> 7 Days): Tracheo-Innominate Fistula

Presentation

This complication is rare, occurring in < 1% of patients.[1] Mortality can be as high as 80%. A tracheo-innominate fistula could potentially be caused by a long tracheostomy tube, usually below the fourth tracheal ring, with high pressure cuff that is too close to the innominate (brachioce-phalic) artery,[2] therefore, causing too much pressure on the innominate artery with subsequent necrosis and erosion of the artery. Other causes include excessive or continuous cuff pressure or neoplastic invasion of the artery. Abnormally high innominate artery could be another contributing factor.

Causes for Rapid Response Activation

Any bleeding at the tracheostomy site should be considered an emergency and rapid response should be activated. Fatal massive bleeding may follow apparently insignificant sentinel bleed in the preceding hours to days of a tracheo-innominate fistula.

Actions

1. Wear protective equipment such as gloves, gown, and face shield or goggles.
2. Maintain continuous pulse oximetry.
3. Maintain continuous cardiac monitoring.
4. Use end tidal CO_2 waveform capnography when available; exhaled carbon dioxide indicates patent or partially patent airway.
5. Apply high flow oxygen to both face and tracheostomy site to maintain SpO_2 > 92% or PaO_2 > 60 mmHg.
6. Look for the chest to rise, listen for breath sounds from the tracheostomy tube, and using your hand, feel for air coming from nose, mouth, or tracheostomy tube.
7. Obtain immediate access to tracheostomy kit.
8. Immediately obtain STAT ENT, anesthesia and cardiothoracic or vascular surgery consultation without delay for investigation.
9. Apply finger pressure to the sternal notch.
10. Slowly and steadily hyperinflate the cuff, if present, with a syringe of air up to 50 mL to tamponade bleeding (avoid rupturing the cuff) and to allow protection from aspiration of blood and to prepare for surgery; this procedure is successful in 85% of cases of tracheo-innominate fistula.[3]
11. If no cuff is present, proceed with oral intubation with cuffed endotracheal tube. While intubating the patient orally, withdraw the tracheostomy tube; place your index finger into the stoma and down the trachea to compress the innominate artery anteriorly against the sternum.

12. Use your thumb in the sternal notch as external pressure, to pinch the innominate artery between your two fingers; maintain this pressure while transporting the patient to the operating room.
13. STAT CBC, coagulation studies, and type and cross.
14. Hold and reverse anticoagulation and correct underlying coagulopathy.
15. Transport the patient to the operating room for ligation and resection of pathological segment of the artery or placement of endovascular stent; surgical intervention may require cardiopulmonary bypass.
16. If patient is stable, angiography by vascular surgeon or interventional radiologist can be done to identify the source of bleeding for subsequent angioembolization.

References

1. Scalise P, Prunk SR, Healy D, Votto J. The incidence of tracheo-arterial fistula in patients with chronic tracheostomy tubes: a retrospective study of 544 patients in a long-term facility. *Chest.* 2005;128:3906–3909.
2. Praveen CV, Martin A. A rare case of fatal hemorrhage after tracheostomy. *Ann R Coll Surg Engl.* 2007;89(8):W6–W8.
3. Jones JW, Reynolds M, Hewitt RL, Drapanas T. Tracheo-innominate artery erosion: successful surgical management of a devastating complication. *Ann Surg.* 1976;184(2):194–204.

Cardiac Catheterization Complication: Hematoma at the Access Site at Common Femoral Artery

Presentation

This is the most common complication of cardiac catheterization. Hematoma is usually formed due to poorly controlled hemostasis post sheath removal. Symptoms and signs include blood oozing from the puncture site, the dressing soaked with blood, or bruising that spreads from the groin to the hip or thigh. Hematoma is usually self-limiting.

Causes for Rapid Response Activation

Large, rapidly expanding hematoma that can lead to hemodynamic instability.

Actions

1. Maintain continuous pulse oximetry.
2. Use supplemental oxygen to maintain $SpO_2 > 92\%$.
3. Maintain continuous cardiac monitoring.
4. Apply manual compression over the artery against the femoral head; 20–30 min of manual compression should result in resolution of hematoma.
5. Stop and reverse all anticoagulation.
6. Place Foley catheter for patients who have urinary retention for urinary bladder decompression.
7. Start IVF resuscitation.
8. Order STAT hemoglobin and hematocrit and transfuse blood if clinically indicated.
9. Assess the affected leg for color, temperature, pedal pulses, and sensation every 15–30 min for 4 h after the bleeding is controlled.
10. Use Doppler ultrasound on the site to rule out pseudoaneurysm or AV fistula.
11. If symptoms fail to resolve, patient will need immediate angiography (a crossover sheath inserted into the contralateral femoral artery and bleeding site localized via angiography) with coiling of the bleeding artery, balloon angioplasty, or graft stent at the site of the vascular trauma.
12. Involve cardiologist who did the procedure early in the course of rapid response.
13. Preventive strategies include use of smaller sheath, early sheath removal, 2–4 h bed rest after removal of sheath, avoidance of venous sheaths, monitoring of heparin doses, and use of vascular closure devices.

Further Reading

1. Tavakol M, Ashraf S, Brener SJ. Risks and complications of coronary angiography: a comprehensive review. *Glob J Health Sci.* 2012;4(1):65–93.

Cardiac Catheterization Complications: Retroperitoneal Hematoma

Presentation

Retroperitoneal bleeding is a potentially life-threatening complication of arterial access, more frequent when the artery is punctured above the inguinal ligament. Usually the bleeding will not be obvious on examination of the access site. Patient will instead experience flank pain, lower back pain, abdominal pain, and leg or flank bruising. Older age and female gender are risk factors.

Causes for Rapid Response Activation

If not recognized early, rapid response can be called due to hemodynamic instability, such as hypotension and tachycardia.

Actions

1. Maintain continuous pulse oximetry.
2. Use supplemental oxygen to maintain $SpO_2 > 92\%$ or $PaO_2 > 60\,mmHg$.
3. Maintain continuous cardiac monitoring.
4. Apply manual compression over the artery against the femoral head; 20–30 min of manual compression should result in resolution of hematoma.
5. Stop and reverse all anticoagulation.
6. Place Foley catheter for patients who have urinary retention for urinary bladder decompression.
7. Start IVF resuscitation.
8. Order STAT hemoglobin and hematocrit and transfuse blood if clinically indicated.
9. Assess the affected leg for color, temperature, pedal pulses, and sensation every 15–30 min for 4 h after the bleeding is controlled.
10. Use Doppler ultrasound on the site to rule out pseudoaneurysm or AV fistula.
11. If symptoms fail to resolve, patient will need tamponade of the puncture site via balloon angioplasty from the ipsilateral or contralateral femoral artery, or immediate angiography with coiling of the bleeding artery.
12. Involve cardiologist who did the procedure early in the course of rapid response.

Further Reading

1. Tavakol M, Ashraf S, Brener SJ. Risks and complications of coronary angiography: a comprehensive review. *Glob J Health Sci.* 2012;4(1):65–93.

Cardiac Catheterization Complications: Contrast-Induced Nephropathy

Presentation

Contrast-induced nephropathy is defined as an elevation of serum creatinine of more than 25% or ≥ 0.5 mg/dL from baseline within 48 h.[1] Contrast agents are based on iodine. According to the National Cardiovascular Data Registry, the incidence of contrast-induced nephropathy was 7.1% among patients undergoing elective and urgent coronary intervention.[2] Patients at higher risk for this complication are those with preexisting chronic kidney disease (creatinine > 1.5 or GFR < 60 mL/min), solitary kidney, congestive heart failure, acute hypotension, diabetes mellitus, over 75 in age, female, and on nephrotoxic medications such as diuretics and ACEI.

Causes for Rapid Response Activation

Chest tightness, hypotension, bradyarrhythmias, acute respiratory failure related to pulmonary congestion.

Actions

1. Maintain continuous pulse oximetry.
2. Use high flow oxygen to maintain SpO_2 > 92%.
3. Maintain continuous cardiac monitoring.
4. Actions are mainly preventative in patients with high risk for contrast nephropathy.
5. Hold nephrotoxic agents such as NSAIDs or loop diuretics 48 h prior to catheterization if possible.
6. Administer isotonic saline (0.9% NaCl) at a rate of 1.0–1.5 mL/kg/h for 3–12 h prior the procedure and continue for 6–24 h after the procedure to maintain urine flow rate of more than 150 mL/h.[3]
7. Use lowest possible volume of a nonionic, low-osmolar iodinated contrast agent, such as iodixanol (Visipaque).
8. No convincing benefit has been found to prescribing oral or intravenous N-acetylcysteine, sodium bicarbonate, or any other pharmacological agents to prevent contrast nephropathy.
9. Delay further exposure to contrast agent until full recovery of renal function, unless benefits of the exposure outweigh the risks.
10. Staging of procedures may help prevent this complication.
11. If despite preventative methods patient still developed pulmonary edema with worsening respiratory status, consult nephrologist for consideration of hemodialysis.

References

1. Mohammed N, Mahfouz A, Achkar A, et al. Contrast induced nephropathy. *Heart Views.* 2013;14(3):106–116.
2. Tsai TT, Patel UD, Chang TI, et al. Contemporary incidence, predictors, and outcomes of acute kidney injury in patients undergoing percutaneous coronary interventions: insights from the NCDR Cath-PCI registry. *JACC Cardiovasc Interv.* 2014;7(1):1–9.
3. Bader BD, Berger ED, Heede MB, et al. What is the best hydration regimen to prevent contrast media-induced nephrotoxicity? *Clin Nephrol.* 2004;62:1–7.

Cardiac Catheterization Complications: Pseudoaneurysm, Arteriovenous Fistula, or Femoral Artery Occlusion

Presentation

Femoral artery pseudoaneurysm is uncommon (0.6%–4.8%)[1]; however, it is a serious complication of cardiac catheterization. Unlike a true aneurysm, which is an excessive dilation of an artery caused by weakness of the arterial wall, a pseudoaneurysm is a leakage of blood from a femoral artery puncture site into the surrounding tissue with a persistent communication between the femoral artery and the adjacent blood collection. It usually occurs between 24 and 48 h after catheterization.[2] Obese patients and patients with atherosclerosis are at high risk. Other risk factors include advanced age, hypertension, low femoral arterial puncture, and large arterial sheath size. Symptoms include groin pain, groin swelling, and lower extremity weakness. Auscultation may reveal a new bruit in the groin area.

Arteriovenous fistula is a direct communication between the arterial and venous puncture sites with ongoing bleeding from the arterial access site that leads to fistula formation. Femoral artery occlusion is rare; however, it must be diagnosed and treated immediately, as delayed treatment can lead to decreased tissue perfusion, ischemia, and loss of limb. A patient with femoral artery occlusion will exhibit what is called the 5 Ps: pain, pallor, paresthesia, pulselessness, and poikilothermia (inability to regulate core body temperature).

Causes for Rapid Response Activation

An enlarging pulsatile hematoma at the puncture site.

Actions

1. Maintain continuous pulse oximetry.
2. Use supplemental oxygen to maintain $SpO_2 > 92\%$.
3. Maintain continuous cardiac monitoring.
4. Order duplex ultrasound to confirm the diagnosis and also to assess the size and origin of the pseudoaneurysm.
5. Treatment options include:
   - Observation of pseudoaneurysm < 2–3 cm in diameter, as it will likely regress spontaneously,[3] followed by serial duplex ultrasound
   - Ultrasound-guided compression
   - Ultrasound-guided thrombin injection has high success rate, even in patients who are being treated with antiplatelets or anticoagulants[4]

    ▪ Surgical endovascular repair for the patients who fail ultrasound-guided compression or ultrasound-guided thrombin injection

6. Consult interventional radiologist early in the course of rapid response.
7. Consult vascular surgeon for surgical repair of the pseudoaneurysm.
8. A follow-up duplex scan is recommended 3–7 days after successful treatment.
9. Arteriovenous fistulas and femoral artery occlusions will require surgical exploration by a vascular surgeon.

References

1. Stone PA, Martinez M, Thompson SN, et al. Ten-year experience of vascular surgeon management of iatrogenic pseudoaneurysms: do anticoagulant and/or antiplatelet medications matter? *Ann Vasc Surg.* 2016;30:45–51.
2. Goldshtein L, Rassin M, Cohen I, Silner D. Critical Care. Managing pseudoaneurysm after cardiac catheterization. *Nursing.* 2006;36(5). 64cc1-64cc2.
3. Kent KC, McArdle CR, Kennedy B, Baim DS, Anninos E, Skillman JJ. A prospective study of the clinical outcome of femoral pseudoaneurysms and arteriovenous fistulas induced by arterial puncture. *J Vasc Surg.* 1993;17(1):125–131.
4. Schneider C, Malisius R, Küchler R, et al. A prospective study on ultrasound-guided percutaneous thrombin injection for treatment of iatrogenic post-catheterisation femoral pseudoaneurysms. *Int J Cardiol.* 2009;131(3):356–361.

Cardiac Catheterization Complications: Anaphylactoid Reactions

Presentation

The incidence of anaphylactoid reactions to contrast media in the catheterization laboratory is 0.23% with one death per 55,000. Contrast media may stimulate histamine, bradykinin, leukotriene, and other mediator release that may cause anaphylactoid reactions. Anaphylactoid reactions usually occur within 20 min of exposure to contrast media.

Symptoms include urticaria, pruritus, bronchospasm, hypotension, and shock.

Causes for Rapid Response Activation

Bronchospasm, hypotension, shock.

Actions

1. Maintain continuous pulse oximetry.
2. Use supplemental oxygen to maintain $SpO_2 > 92\%$.
3. Maintain continuous cardiac monitoring.
4. Management of urticaria and pruritus:
   - Diphenhydramine 25–50 mg IV

   If no improvement:
   - Epinephrine 0.3 mL of 1:1000 solution subcutaneously q 15 min, up to 1 mL
   - Cimetidine 300 mg IV over 15 min
5. Management of bronchospasm:
   - Epinephrine 0.3 mL of 1:1000 solution subcutaneously q 15 min, up to 1 mL
   - Continuous albuterol nebulizer 0.2 mg/L
   - Diphenhydramine 25–50 mg IV
   - Cimetidine 300 mg IV over 15 min
   - Hydrocortisone 200–400 mg IV
6. Management of facial/laryngeal edema:
   - Assess airway and intubate if indicated; consult anesthesiologist if patient has difficult airway
   - Epinephrine 0.3 mL of 1:1000 solution subcutaneously q 15 min, up to 1 mL
   - Diphenhydramine 25–50 mg IV
   - Cimetidine 300 mg IV over 15 min
   - Hydrocortisone 200–400 mg IV

7. Management of hypotension/shock:
   - Assess airway and intubate if indicated; consult anesthesiologist especially if patient has difficult airway
   - Epinephrine 10 μg/min IV until target blood pressure response; then 1–4 μg/min to maintain target blood pressure
   - Fluid resuscitation: 1–3 L of 0.9% saline within first hour
   - Diphenhydramine 50–100 mg IV
   - Cimetidine 300 mg IV over 15 min
   - Hydrocortisone 200–400 mg IV
   - If refractory to epinephrine drip, add dopamine drip at 2–15 μg/kg/min
8. Pretreatment with antihistamines and corticosteroids and use of iso-osmolar agents may decrease the risk of anaphylactoid reactions.

Further Reading

1. Goss JE, Chambers CE, Heupler FA, et al. Systemic anaphylactoid reactions to iodinated contrast media during cardiac catheterization procedures: guidelines for prevention, diagnosis and treatment. *CathLabDigest.* 2006;14(9).

Paracentesis Complications: Paracentesis-Induced Circulatory Dysfunction

Presentation

This complication usually occurs following large volume (> 5 L) paracentesis.[1] Large volume of fluid shifts back to peritoneum causing reaccumulation of ascites and decreases intravascular fluid volume. Incidence is 15%–30% when large volume paracentesis is performed with plasma volume expanders such as albumin.[1] Patients will develop recurring abdominal distention, abdominal pain, and shortness of breath. This complication is associated with higher mortality, as patients may develop hyponatremia and hepatorenal syndrome.

Causes for Rapid Response Activation

Progressively worsening dyspnea or hypotension.

Actions

1. Maintain continuous pulse oximetry.
2. Use supplemental oxygen to maintain SpO_2 > 92%.
3. Maintain continuous cardiac monitoring.
4. Prevention:
   - Albumin 6–8 g/L of ascitic fluid removed for large volume (> 5 L) paracentesis[2]; for example, if 7 L of ascites removed, administer 25% albumin 42–56 g IV during or immediately after paracentesis.
   - Avoid large volume paracentesis in hemodynamically unstable patients.
5. Treatment:
   - Hold diuretics and β-blockers.
   - Albumin 6–8 g/L of ascitic fluid removed for large volume (> 5 L) paracentesis[2]; for example, if 7 L of ascites removed, administer 25% albumin 42–56 g IV.

References

1. Lindsay AJ, Burton J, Ray CE. Paracentesis induced circulatory dysfunction: a primer for the interventional radiologist. *Semin Intervent Radiol.* 2014;31(3):276–278.
2. Runyon BA. Introduction to the revised American Association for the Study of Liver Diseases Practice Guideline management of adult patients with ascites due to cirrhosis 2012. *Hepatology.* 2013;57:1651–1653.

Paracentesis Complications: Persistent Leakage of Ascitic Fluid From Puncture Site

Presentation

Another complication of paracentesis is a 5% risk of ascitic fluid leakage in patients undergoing large volume (> 5 L) paracentesis.[1] Usually this complication is self-limited. Persistent leakage is associated with increased morbidity.

Actions

1. Prevention:
   - Use Z-track. While inserting the needle into peritoneal cavity, pull the skin 2 cm caudally with nondominant hand.
   - Insert the needle at 45° angle.
2. Initial treatment:
   - Place 4×4 cm sterile dressing on the site of the puncture.
   - Lay the patient on the side opposite the puncture site for 2–6 h to reduce pressure on the clot and to reduce disruption of the clot.
   - If dressing becomes saturated, remove it and place an ostomy bag over the site of leakage until it seals off; ostomy bag will keep the leaking fluid contained, prevent the skin from irritation by ascitic fluid, and monitor the quantity of the leakage.
   - Place a single suture to close the skin.
3. If ascitic leak is persistent and refractory to conservative treatment, consider the following:
   - Autologous blood patch: 30 mL of the patient's peripheral blood is injected adjacent to the site of the ascitic leakage with subsequent obliteration of the paracentesis tract.[2]
   - Perform surgical abdominal wall layer closure.

References

1. De Gottardi A, Thévenot T, Spahr L, et al. Risk of complications after abdominal paracentesis in cirrhotic patients: a prospective study. *Clin Gastroenterol Hepatol.* 2009;7:906–909.
2. Khan N, Dushay KM. Autologous blood patch for persistent ascites leak from non-closing paracentesis tracts. *Med Sci.* 2019;7(9):88.

Paracentesis Complications: Hemorrhage

Presentation

Abdominal wall hematoma (more common) and hemoperitoneum (less common) can complicate 1% of paracentesis cases and can occur within minutes to days after a procedure.[1] Patients with severe liver disease with MELD score > 25 are at higher risk. Risk is higher in patients with INR > 1.6, PT > 21 s and platelet count $< 50,000/mm^3$.[2] The prognosis for these patients is poor, with a 30-day mortality of 42.6%.[3] The most common source of bleeding is the inferior epigastric artery.[3] An abdominal wall hematoma can manifest as a tender bruise around a puncture site and can be assessed by ultrasound. Hemoperitoneum may manifest as hemorrhagic ascites, causing abdominal distention and pain. Rarely patients with hemoperitoneum can develop hypovolemia or acute kidney injury.

Causes for Rapid Response Activation

Hypotension, tachycardia, pallor.

Actions

1. Maintain continuous pulse oximetry.
2. Use supplemental oxygen to maintain $SpO_2 > 92\%$.
3. Maintain continuous cardiac monitoring.
4. Labs: CBC (anemia, thrombocytopenia) and coagulation studies (PT/INR).[3]
5. Perform diagnostic paracentesis to assess the presence of visible blood.[3]
6. If diagnostic paracentesis confirms presence of blood in peritoneal fluid, a CT scan of the abdomen/pelvis should be done.[3]
7. If CT scan of abdomen/pelvis is inconclusive, consider angiography.[3]
8. Start supportive treatment with IV fluids such as normal saline and IV albumin.[3]
9. Transfuse blood products such as packed red blood cells, platelets, and fresh frozen plasma as indicated.[3]
10. Consult interventional radiologist for transcatheter coiling and embolization of inferior epigastric artery.[3]
11. Consult general surgeon for consideration of surgical drainage of abdominal wall hematomas, laparoscopy or laparotomy with ligation of the bleeding artery, and TIPS (transjugular intrahepatic portosystemic shunting).[3]

12. Prevention:
  - Practice guidelines from the American Association for the Study of Liver Diseases (AASLD), the International Ascites Club, and the European Association for the Study of the Liver (EASL) do not consider paracentesis to be unsafe in the presence of marked thrombocytopenia or prolongation in the prothrombin time, nor do they recommend correction of these parameters prior to paracentesis.[3]
  - Avoid rectus abdominis muscle due to proximity of large epigastric arteries.
  - Avoid surgical scars due to potential neovascularization and engorged subcutaneous veins.
  - Use linear vascular ultrasound probe to better assess subcutaneous vessels.

References

1. De Gottardi A, Thévenot T, Spahr L, et al. Risk of complications after abdominal paracentesis in cirrhotic patients: a prospective study. *Clin Gastroenterol Hepatol.* 2009;7:906–909.
2. Gines P, Cardenas A, Rodes J. Management of cirrhosis and ascites. *N Engl J Med.* 2004;350(16):1646–1654.
3. Katz MJ, Sharzehi K, Jain V, Naveed A, et al. Hemorrhagic complications of paracentesis: a systematic review of the literature. *Gastroenterol Res Pract.* 2014; 2014:985141.

Paracentesis Complications: Visceral Perforation (Bladder, Stomach, Bowel)

Presentation

Incidence is <0.5% cases.[1] Perforation is less common with diagnostic than with therapeutic paracentesis. Most perforations cause self-limited peritonitis that does not require surgical intervention. Patients with distended bladder due to medications or a medical condition are at higher risk for bladder perforation.

Symptoms of visceral perforation include fever, chills, sweating, nausea, vomiting, worsening abdominal distention, and pain. Patients with bladder perforation will have gross hematuria, difficulty urinating, inability to void, and suprapubic pain or tenderness.

Examination of patient will show signs of acute abdomen, such as absent bowel sounds, guarding, and rebound tenderness.

Causes for Rapid Response Activation

Tachycardia, tachypnea, hypotension.

Actions

1. Maintain continuous pulse oximetry.
2. Use supplemental oxygen to maintain SpO_2 >92%.
3. Maintain continuous cardiac monitoring.
4. Labs: CBC (low hemoglobin, leukocytosis), and CMP (electrolytes, creatinine, metabolic acidosis, transaminases); urinalysis in patients with bladder perforation will show gross or microscopic hematuria; consider blood cultures.
5. Order bowel rest.
6. Plain supine and erect abdominal X-ray will show free intraperitoneal air.
7. CT abdomen and pelvis with water-soluble oral contrast will demonstrate free intraperitoneal air, increased amount of peritoneal fluid, and also will be useful in localization of perforation.
8. CT cystography in patients with suspected bladder perforation will detect even subtle perforation.
9. Start aggressive IV fluid resuscitation.
10. Correct electrolytes.
11. Administer broad-spectrum IV antibiotics to cover anaerobes and gram-negative bacteria[2]:
    - Metronidazole 1 g IV loading dose, followed by 500 mg IV every 6 h[3] and cefepime 2 g IV q 12 h[4] for 7–10 days
    - Piperacillin/tazobactam 3.375 g IV q 6 h[5] for 7–10 days

12. Consult urologist for consideration of surgical repair of bladder perforation, if indicated.
13. Consult general surgeon for consideration of laparoscopic or open surgical repair of gastric or intestinal perforation, if indicated.[5]
14. Prevention:
    - Avoid surgical scars where potential adhesions could be.
    - Use ultrasound to identify the deepest pocket of at least 3 cm.
    - Empty bladder by voiding or catheterization before paracentesis to avoid puncture.

References

1. De Gottardi A, Thévenot T, Spahr L, et al. Risk of complications after abdominal paracentesis in cirrhotic patients: a prospective study. *Clin Gastroenterol Hepatol.* 2009;7:906–909.
2. Melmer PD, Banks T, Holmes S, Sciarretta JD, Davis JM. Gastroduodenal surgery: a persistent and continuing challenge. *Am Surg.* 2018;84(7):1204–1206.
3. *Metronidazole.* Reference.medscape.com.
4. *Cefepime.* Reference.medscape.com.
5. *Piperacillin/Tazobactam.* Reference.medscape.com.

Complications of Thoracentesis: Pneumothorax

Presentation

Iatrogenic pneumothorax is the most common complication of thoracentesis. A systematic review and metaanalysis of 24 studies, including a total of 6605 cases that received thoracentesis, reported an overall 6.0% incidence of pneumothorax.[1] A more recent study of 9320 thoracentesis in 4618 patients reported a 0.61% incidence of thoracentesis-related pneumothorax.[2]

Risk for iatrogenic pneumothorax is higher in therapeutic thoracentesis, in mechanically ventilated patients, and in two or more needle insertions. Chest tube placement may be required in up to 50% of cases, with a mean duration of placement of approximately 4 days.[1]

The incidence of iatrogenic pneumothorax can be reduced by real-time ultrasonography use. Experienced operators may have lower pneumothorax rates.[1]

Symptomatic patients may experience stabbing chest pain that may radiate to ipsilateral shoulder and worsen with inspiration, dyspnea, cough, and diaphoresis. On physical examination, patients may have tachypnea and distant or absent breath sounds on affected side.

Causes for Rapid Response Activation

Chest pain, dyspnea, tachypnea, tachycardia.

Actions

1. Maintain continuous pulse oximetry.
2. Use supplemental oxygen to maintain $SpO_2 > 90\%$ or $PaO_2 > 60\,mmHg$.
3. Maintain continuous cardiac monitoring.
4. Unstable patients should be treated with needle aspiration: place a large-bore 14–16 gauge and 4.5 cm in length angiocatheter superior to the rib, in the second intercostal space in the midclavicular line, as a temporary measure.[3]
5. Labs: ABG; treatment should not be delayed while awaiting the results; may be useful to evaluate the severity of hypoxia, hypercarbia, and respiratory acidosis.[4]
6. Order chest X-ray, not for confirmation of the diagnosis, but when patient is stable, to assess extent of pneumothorax and potential causes.[4]
7. Perform bedside ultrasonography for hemodynamically unstable patients.[4]
8. In patients with primary spontaneous pneumothorax:
   - If pneumothorax is < 15% and patient is asymptomatic, treatment of choice is observation and administration of 100% oxygen to promote resolution.
   - If pneumothorax is < 15% and patient is symptomatic, needle aspiration is treatment of choice.
   - If pneumothorax is > 15%, treatment of choice is aspiration with pigtail catheter, left to low suction, or water seal.[4]

9. Patients with parenchymal lung disease with chronic pulmonary conditions such as asthma, COPD, cystic fibrosis, sarcoidosis, bronchogenic carcinoma, idiopathic pulmonary fibrosis, or pulmonary TB may need tube thoracostomy.[4]

References

1. Gordon CE, Feller-Kopman D, Balk EM, et al. Pneumothorax following thoracentesis. A systematic review and meta-analysis. *Arch Intern Med.* 2010;170(4):332–339.
2. Ault MJ, Rosen BT, Scher J, et al. Thoracentesis outcomes: a 12-year experience. *Thorax.* 2015;70:127–132.
3. McKnight CL, Burns B. Pneumothorax. StatPearls Publishing Ncbi.nim.nih.gov. Updated: November 16, 2020.
4. Daley BJ, Bhimji S, Bascom R, Benninghoff MG, Alam S. *Pneumothorax treatment and management.* April 28, 2020 Emedicine.medscape.com.

Complications of Thoracentesis: Hemothorax

Presentation

The incidence of iatrogenic hemothorax after thoracentesis is estimated to be around 0.1%.[1] It usually occurs within 24 h after thoracentesis.[1] Usually, hemorrhage results from injury to the intercostal artery during needle access. The intercostal artery can be tortuous and does not always lie along the inferior rib edge. Risk of bleeding can be significantly decreased by the use of color Doppler US for guidance of thoracentesis.[1]

Symptomatic patients might experience stabbing chest pain that may radiate to the ipsilateral shoulder and worsen with inspiration, dyspnea, cough, and diaphoresis. On physical examination, patients may have tachypnea and distant or absent breath sounds on affected side.

Causes for Rapid Response Activation

Chest pain, dyspnea, tachypnea, tachycardia, hypotension.

Actions

1. Maintain continuous pulse oximetry.
2. Use supplemental oxygen to maintain $SpO_2 > 90\%$ or $PaO_2 > 60\,mmHg$.
3. Maintain continuous cardiac monitoring.
4. Labs: CBC (anemia, low platelets) and coagulation studies (elevated INR).
5. Upright chest radiograph will confirm diagnosis by demonstration of costophrenic angle blunting by meniscus of fluid; if the patient is unable to stand, a portable supine chest radiograph may show apical capping of fluid surrounding the superior pole of the lung.[2]
6. Bedside ultrasonography may be used for hemodynamically unstable patients.
7. Chest CT will detect hemothorax as hyperattenuating (35–70 Hounsfield units) effusion with dependent layering of dense clots.[1]
8. In hypotensive patients, place a large-bore IV line and start IV fluid resuscitation at 20 mL/kg of normal saline or lactated Ringer solution.
9. Transfuse blood as necessary.
10. Tube thoracostomy is the treatment of choice; usually in the sixth or seventh intercostal space at the posterior axillary line; patients with hemopneumothorax may need placement of two chest tubes, with the tube draining the pneumothorax placed in a more superior and anterior position.[2]
11. Repeat chest X-ray after placement of chest tube to visualize the position of the chest tube and to assess the degree of hemothorax evacuation.[2]
12. Put chest tube to water seal after the lung is fully reexpanded on chest X-ray, fluid drainage is < 50 mL/24 h, and no significant residual air leak is present.[2]
13. In case of persistent bleeding, consult cardiovascular surgeon for consideration of thoracotomy.[2]

References

1. Massimo T. *Iatrogenic Haemothorax Following Thoracentesis*; 2018. Eurorad.org.
2. Mancini MC. *Hemothorax*. Updated July 13, 2020 Emedicine.medscape.com.

Complications of Thoracentesis: Infection/Empyema

Presentation

Iatrogenic empyema is a rare complication of thoracentesis. It is defined as collection of pus in the pleural cavity as a result of inoculation of pleural space during or after thoracentesis. Mortality is estimated to be around 6%–24%.[1] Elderly patients, patients with chronic comorbidities, immunocompromised patients, and patients with malignancies have higher mortality rates. Hospital-associated bacteria such as MRSA, *Pseudomonas aeruginosa*, and anaerobic bacteria are implicated in the pathophysiology of iatrogenic empyema.

Symptoms include fever, chills, sweating, cough, shortness of breath, and pleuritic chest pain. On physical examination, patients may have tachypnea, rales, rhonchi, and diminished breath sounds.

Causes for Rapid Response Activation

Progressively worsening dyspnea, tachypnea, hypoxia, altered mental status.

Actions

1. Maintain continuous pulse oximetry.
2. Use supplemental oxygen to maintain $SpO_2 > 90\%$ or $PaO_2 > 60\,mmHg$.
3. Maintain continuous cardiac monitoring.
4. Labs: CBC (leukocytosis, left shift, bandemia, low platelets), CMP (assess concomitant electrolyte abnormalities or elevated creatinine), procalcitonin (elevated in bacterial infection), and ABG.
5. Order sputum, pleural fluid and blood cultures.
6. Chest X-ray (standard 2-view) may demonstrate obliterated costophrenic angle, extension of the air-fluid level to the chest wall, extension of air-fluid level across fissure lines, and a tapering border of the air-fluid collection.[2]
7. Chest CT scan has increased sensitivity in detection of pulmonary infection compared to chest X-ray, especially in immunocompromised patients.[2]
8. Empirical antibiotic therapy should be guided by local resistance patterns; however, it generally should cover hospital-acquired pathogens such as MRSA, *Pseudomonas aeruginosa*, and anaerobic bacteria:
   - Vancomycin 15 mg/kg IV every 12 h[3] (adjust the dose based on trough levels) and Piperacillin/tazobactam 4.5 g IV every 6 h[4]
9. Antibiotics should be deescalated based on pleural cultures and sensitivities.
10. A CT-guided or US-guided pigtail drainage catheter is not inferior to a large caliber thoracostomy tube and causes much less pain.[5]

11. If refractory to treatment, consider intrapleural fibrinolysis with streptokinase.[6]
12. If refractory to all above treatments, consult cardiothoracic surgeon for video-assisted thoracic surgery (VATS).[6]

References

1. Ahmed AE, Yacoub TE. Empyema thoracis. *Clin Med Insights Circ Respir Pulm Med.* 2010;4:1–8.
2. Tobler M. *Empyema Imaging.* Emedicine.medscape.com. Updated: October 28, 2019.
3. *Vancomycin (Rx).* Reference.medscape.com.
4. *Piperacillin/Tazobactam (Rx).* Reference.medscape.com.
5. Hyeon Y. Management of pleural effusion, empyema, and lung abscess. *Semin Intervent Radiol.* 2011;28(1):75–86.
6. Ward MA. *Empyema and Abscess.* Emedicine.medscape.com. Updated: March 15, 2018.

Complications of Thoracentesis: Liver/Spleen Injury

Presentation

Liver and spleen injuries are rare complications of right-sided and left-sided thoracentesis and generally resolve spontaneously. Diagnostic ultrasound helps to guide treatment of these complications. In hepatic injuries, patients may experience right upper quadrant pain with radiation to the right shoulder due to diaphragmatic irritation. In spleen injuries, patients may experience left upper quadrant pain with radiation to the left shoulder due to diaphragmatic irritation.

Causes for Rapid Response Activation

Staff member has significant concern about the patient's condition.

Actions

1. Labs: CBC (baseline Hg), CMP (baseline transaminases), and coagulation studies (INR, PT, aPTT).
2. CT scan of abdomen with IV contrast is the imaging of choice; in hepatic injuries, it may demonstrate a hematoma as well-defined hypodensity between the liver and its capsule in the area of the puncture site; in a splenic injury, it may demonstrate a small subcapsular or intraparenchymal hematoma.
3. Monitor with serial physical examinations, labs, and ultrasounds for 24–48 h.
4. Most intrahepatic and splenic hematomas resolve spontaneously without surgical intervention.

Further Reading

1. Shah C, Johnson PT. *Iatrogenic Liver Hematoma.* SonoWorld.com.
2. Bjerke HS. *Splenic Rupture.* Emedicine.medscape.com. Updated: April 3, 2017.

Complications of Lumbar Puncture: Post-LP Headache

Presentation

Headaches are common complications of lumbar puncture and occur in 32% of patients,[1] due to a small amount of CSF leakage from the dura at the needle insertion site. The onset of headaches occurs within 24–28 h after the procedure. The headache is usually located in the frontal and occipital areas and is postural. It is alleviated in a flat position and worsened in an upright position. Other symptoms include dizziness, tinnitus, visual changes, photophobia, nausea, vomiting, neck pain, and stiffness. Although rare, if the leak becomes persistent, the headaches may become severe and immobilize the patient. This condition is usually self-limiting and resolves within 48 h, more rarely within 7 days.[2]

Post-LP headaches can be prevented by the use of bedside ultrasonography for identification of pertinent landmarks, a lateral decubitus position, and a less traumatic type of LP needle, such as a pencil-point needle with a smaller gauge, rather than a sharp or cutting needle with a larger-gauge (≤ 22 gauge).[3]

Causes for Rapid Response Activation

Severe headache, visual changes, dizziness.

Actions

1. Have patient lie flat.
2. Obtain vitals.
3. Use supplemental oxygen to maintain $SpO_2 > 92\%$.
4. Administer IV fluid hydration; avoid fluid overload.
5. Administer analgesics: acetaminophen and/or ibuprofen.
6. Administer caffeine 250–500 mg IV every 6 h (no consistent evidence).[2]
7. Rarely headaches can be due to post-LP subdural hematoma; if headaches do not improve with bedrest and adequate IV fluids, perform head CT scan to rule out subdural hematoma.
8. Consult anesthesiologist for epidural blood patch for severe headaches.[2]

References

1. Ahmed SV, Jayawarna C, Jude E. Post lumbar puncture headache: diagnosis and management. *Postgrad Med J.* 2006;82(973):713–716.
2. Shlamovitz GZ. *Lumbar Puncture.* Emedicine.medscape.com. Updated: September 8, 2020.
3. *Lumbar Puncture – Reducing the Risk of Post-Procedure Headache.* Spinal CSF leak foundation; 2017. Spinalcsfleak.org.

Complications of Lumbar Puncture: Spinal Hematoma

Presentation

Although spinal hematoma is a very rare complication of lumbar puncture or neuraxial anesthesia, it can have a detrimental outcome, especially in patients with a suboptimum coagulation state. Approximately 4% of symptomatic spinal hematomas are related to lumbar puncture.[1] Spinal hematomas are mostly epidural, whereas subarachnoid and subdural hematomas occur in less than 20% of cases.[1] Spinal hematoma usually occurs within 24–48 h after the procedure.[2]

Patients with coagulopathies (liver disorder, alcoholism, thrombocytopenia), anticoagulant therapy, vascular malformations, and immunocompromised status are at higher risk for spinal hematoma after a lumbar puncture.[1] Use of thromboprophylaxis in patients who receive epidural anesthesia for knee arthroplasty is another example of increased risk for spinal hematoma.

Symptoms may include severe acute back pain that worsens with coughing, sneezing, or straining; lower extremity pain; numbness in lower extremities; and paraparesis that can progress to paraplegia and bowel and bladder incontinence in severe cases.

Spinal hematomas can be prevented by avoiding lumbar puncture or neuraxial anesthesia in patients who are on anticoagulant therapy, have received thrombolytic therapy, or have coagulopathies.

Causes for Rapid Response Activation

Progressively worsening neurological compromise.

Actions

1. Consult neurosurgeon as soon as spinal hematoma is suspected, as diagnostic work-up, such as a spinal MRI, will take time.
2. Labs: CBC (anemia), CMP (concomitant electrolyte abnormalities, elevated creatinine, elevated transaminases), and coagulation studies (INR, PT, aPTT).
3. A whole-spine MRI with and without gadolinium is the imaging of choice and will show hematoma compressing spinal cord or cauda equina; will also show location, extent, and age of hematoma and degree of cord compression.[1,2]
4. Correct clotting abnormalities immediately, if present.
5. High-dose steroid therapy does not contribute to improved neurologic recovery but will increase adverse effects, such as hyperglycemia and pneumonia, in patients with an acute spinal cord injury.[3,4]
6. Neurosurgeon will decide whether to observe or operate.[2]
7. Patients with hematomas localized at the cauda equina level with minimal neurologic symptoms without motor deficits can be observed.[2]
8. Surgical management, such as emergent decompressive laminectomy with evacuation of spinal hematoma, is indicated for patients with rapidly progressing neurologic deficits.[1,2]

References

1. Jishi AA, Murty N. Massive lumbar spine hematoma post-spinal tap. *Surg Neurol Int.* 2017;8:293.
2. Nelson A, Benzon HT, Jabri RS. *Diagnosis and Management of Spinal and Peripheral Nerve Hematoma.* Nysora.com.
3. Liu Z, Yang Y, He L, et al. High-dose methylprednisolone for acute traumatic spinal cord injury. A meta-analysis. *Neurology.* 2019;93(9).
4. Sultan I, Lamba N, Liew A, et al. The safety and efficacy of steroid treatment for acute spinal cord injury: a systematic review and meta-analysis. *Heliyon.* 2020;6(2), e03414.

Complications of Lumbar Puncture: Cerebral Herniation

Presentation

Cerebral herniation is a rare complication of lumbar puncture with an incidence of 0.1%–3%.[1] It usually occurs within 24 h after lumbar puncture.[2] The outcome is often fatal.

A preprocedure noncontrast CT scan of head should be done in patients with suspicion of elevated intracranial pressure, for example, due to a mass or space-occupying lesion. A decreasing level of consciousness with a Glasgow Coma Scale (GSC) ≤ 11, a recent seizure, brainstem signs such as evidence of cranial nerve palsies (pupillary changes), and posturing or irregular respirations should be indications for delaying lumbar puncture even in the setting of a normal CT scan of head.[3]

Symptoms of herniation may include lower extremity weakness, anisocoria with fixed dilated pupil, posturing with loss of brainstem reflexes, irregular respiration, and respiratory arrest.

Causes for Rapid Response Activation

Rapidly progressing neurological deterioration.

Actions

1. Maintain continuous pulse oximetry.
2. Use supplemental oxygen to maintain $SpO_2 \geq 94\%$ or $PaO_2 > 100$ mmHg.
3. Maintain continuous cardiac monitoring and blood pressure measurements.
4. Consult neurosurgeon emergently.
5. Elevate head of bed to 15–30 degrees; this is associated with a significant decrease in ICP and assure neutral and midline position of the head to keep jugular veins open.
6. Control pain with opioid analgesics, for example, IV morphine, as pain can increase intracranial pressure.
7. Control agitation with benzodiazepines, for example, IV lorazepam, as agitation can increase intracranial pressure.
8. Control fever with antipyretics such as rectal acetaminophen and cooling blankets.
9. Control hypertension with medications that reduce systemic hypertension without affecting ICP and with short half-life, for example:
   - Administer esmolol loading dose 500 µg/kg IV over 1 min, followed by 50 µg/kg/min; titrate to maximum of 200 µg/kg/min.[4]
   - Administer labetalol 20 mg IV bolus; may repeat doses of 20–80 mg IV at 10 min intervals until goal blood pressure is achieved, with a maximum 24 h total of 300 mg[4]; dose reduction may be needed in hepatic impairment.
10. Treat seizures or nonconvulsive status with antiepileptics.

11. Consult neurosurgery for ventricular catheter placement through a burr hole to monitor ICP; the catheter should be checked for proper functioning every 2–4 h and anytime there is a change in the ICP, CSF output, or neurological exam.[5]

12. Administer mannitol as an initial bolus of 0.25–1 g/kg IV; this can be repeated at 0.25–0.5 g/kg IV doses every 6–8 h as needed; renal toxicity is one of the primary concerns therefore check serum osmolarity to calculate osmolar gap (osmolar gap = measured serum osmolarity − calculated serum osmolarity); goal osmolar gap is < 18–20; other concerns include extravasation and fluid-electrolyte imbalance.[6]

13. Administer IV fluids such as crystalloids to maintain euvolemia, as mannitol may cause urinary osmotic diuresis and decrease plasma osmolarity.

14. Neurosurgeon may consider decompressive craniectomy if the previously mentioned strategies do not improve patient's condition.

References

1. McDowell KE, Chapman AL. Cerebral herniation after lumbar puncture. *Clin Infect Dis.* 2019;69(7):1266–1267.

2. Hasbun R. *When Is Cerebral Herniation Most Likely to Occur Following Lumbar Puncture (LP) for Meningitis?* . Emedicine.medscape.com. Updated: July 16, 2019.

3. Joffe AR. Lumbar puncture and brain herniation in acute bacterial meningitis: a review. *J Intensive Care Med.* 2007;22(4):194–207.

4. Levy ZD, Zhou Q, Slesinger TL. Hypertensive crises. In: *Critical Care Emergency Medicine.* 2nd ed. McGrawHill Education; vol. 17; 2017:175–183.

5. Rangel-Castillo L, Gopinath S, Robertson CS. Management of Intracranial Hypertension. *Neurol Clin.* 2008;26(2):521–541.

6. Multum C. *Mannitol.* Drugs.com. Medically reviewed on September 23, 2020.

CHAPTER 10

Rapid Response Cases

Case I

Forty-four-year-old obese male with BMI of 40, with diabetes mellitus type II with the last HgA1C of 9 about 2 months ago, with HTN, and who smokes and has sedentary lifestyle made a New Year's resolution to start a weight loss program. Unfortunately, during his first session in the gym, while doing jumping jacks, he landed on an inverted left foot and developed a sprain in his left ankle.

Patient treated the ankle sprain with rest, ice, compression, and elevation; however, about 3–4 days after the injury, he developed progressively worsening ankle pain, redness, and swelling over the lateral aspect of the left ankle that continued to spread up the left lower extremity to below the knee level. Patient also developed fever of 101.3, at which point he presented to emergency department and was admitted to the acute care ward.

On physical examination in the acute care ward, patient's left lower extremity was erythematous, edematous, warm, and tender to touch. Patient had diminished dorsalis pedis pulse.

Patient was diagnosed with left lower extremity acute cellulitis and was started on IV fluids, IV cefazolin, and correctional insulin sliding scale. His home medications for DM and HTN were continued. He was started on enoxaparin 40 mg subcutaneously daily for pharmacological VTE prophylaxis. Doppler US of the left lower extremity did not show evidence of DVT. His left leg was elevated.

Patient was slowly improving in terms of his left lower extremity cellulitis; however, about 3 days after admission, he suddenly developed progressively worsening shortness of breath and chest pain with deep breaths. Nursing staff proceeded with obtaining vital signs, which were remarkable for tachycardia of 115 and hypotension of 80/50, and rapid response was activated.

On examination, patient was found to be in moderate distress due to dyspnea, heart auscultation was remarkable for tachycardia, and lung auscultation was remarkable for tachypnea. Repeat heart rate was 120 and repeat blood pressure was 75/40. Patient was started on norepinephrine drip at 10 µg/min IV infusion. Stat EKG showed sinus tachycardia with HR of 126. Stat bedside echo showed dilated RV with septal shift. Patient was started on heparin drip with bolus of 80 U/kg, followed by 18 U/kg/h. With norepinephrine drip, patient's blood pressure improved to 100/60. As patient was now hemodynamically stable, CT angiogram of chest was done and confirmed a large filling defect over the bifurcation of the pulmonary artery, exhibiting "a saddle embolus." A checklist of contraindications for systemic thrombolysis did not reveal any contraindications. Heparin drip was held. Patient was treated with alteplase 100 mg IV over 2 h without any complications. After completion of alteplase, aPTT was checked and was found to be 75 s (< 80 s). Heparin drip was restarted at 18 U/kg/h. Patient was started on warfarin, and when INR was therapeutic at 2.7 for 48 h, heparin drip was discontinued and patient was discharged home on warfarin for 3 months.

Debriefing

All team members agreed that communication between team members was clear and effective. All team members understood their roles and responsibilities. Situational awareness was appropriately maintained. Workload was distributed efficiently. Assistance was asked for and offered when needed. No errors were identified; however, it was recommended to the patient's attending physician and pharmacist to use weight-based dosing of enoxaparin for adequate pharmacological VTE prophylaxis in morbidly obese patients; for example, this patient's enoxaparin was supposed to be dosed at 40 mg SC q 12 h.

Case II

Seventy-four-year-old female patient with mild dementia, HTN, and malnourishment of unknown etiology presented to emergency department with 4-day history of fever, malaise, cough, shortness of breath, and decreased oral intake. Diagnostic work-up was remarkable for leukocytosis with left shift, elevated procalcitonin, and right lower lobe infiltrate on chest X-ray. She was diagnosed with pneumonia and was started on antibiotic treatment for pneumonia.

As patient also had hypokalemia secondary to poor oral intake, potassium chloride 40 mEq orally was ordered. While trying to swallow the potassium pill, patient developed sudden onset of cough and gaging. Patient's nurse activated rapid response call.

Medical resident, who responded first to the rapid response call, assessed the patient, who continued to cough and gag but was able to vocalize. Vital signs were stable with SpO_2 94%. On physical examination, patient had wheezing. Medical resident performed Heimlich maneuver, during which patient became aphonic, was no longer able to breathe, and subsequently became unconscious. SpO_2 decreased to 74%.

Respiratory therapist, who had responded by this time, lowered the patient to the ground and started CPR. Bag-mask ventilation was avoided to prevent the pill from potentially moving below the vocal cords. At that point, hospitalist who had arrived at patient's room performed direct laryngoscopy and was able to visualize and remove the potassium pill using Magill forceps. With bag-mask ventilation, patient's oxygenation improved, she regained consciousness, and started to breathe on her own. Vital signs were normal with SpO_2 96%.

Debriefing

All team members agreed that communication between team members was clear and effective. All team members understood their roles and responsibilities. Situational awareness was appropriately maintained. Workload was distributed efficiently. Assistance was asked for and offered when needed.

The medical resident was educated about the management of partial and complete upper airway obstruction and how important it is to avoid Heimlich maneuver in patients who are able to vocalize and protect their airway. It was recommended to the patient's attending physician to keep the patient NPO with aspiration precautions and order a speech therapist evaluation for swallowing and recommendations on diet and pill administration.

Case III

Fifty-seven-year-old female underwent cardiac catheterization through right femoral access. Femoral access was chosen over the radial access due to extensive peripheral arterial disease. Shortly after arrival from the catheterization lab to patient's room, the nurse noticed blood oozing from the puncture site. She activated rapid response call and applied direct pressure to the puncture site. Vital signs were done by the nurse's assistant and were found to be normal.

Hospitalist who responded to rapid response activation assessed patient's lower extremities, which were found to have normal color, temperature, diminished pedal pulses which is the patient's baseline, and normal sensation to touch. Hospitalist ordered hemoglobin and coagulation studies (INR, PT, aPTT). After 25 min of manual compression over the artery against the femoral head, bleeding completely resolved.

Debriefing

All team members agreed that communication between team members was clear and effective. All team members understood their roles and responsibilities. Situational awareness was appropriately maintained. Workload was distributed efficiently. Assistance was asked for and offered when needed. No errors were identified.

Case IV

Seventy-two-year-old male without any past medical history presented to emergency department with 2-day history of progressively worsening right upper quadrant pain. Pain had been intermittent and was worse with eating. The day of presentation, patient also experienced fever and chills. Diagnostic work-up was remarkable for elevated white blood cell count and total bilirubin. CT scan of abdomen/pelvis with IV contrast was ordered by the resident in order to assess for acute cholecystitis. Patient reported no prior history of allergies.

About 10 min after IV iodinated contrast medium was injected, patient developed sudden onset of flushing, nausea, and dizziness. Vitals signs were done, and patient was found to have SpO_2 of 88%, HR of 46, and blood pressure of 85/40. On lung auscultation, patient was found to have wheezing. Rapid response was activated by the nurse. Continuous pulse oximetry and cardiac monitoring were started. Patient was started on oxygen at 10–12 L/min via a partial nonrebreathing mask. Patient's lower extremities were elevated.

The resident who ordered the CT scan immediately arrived at the scene and assessed the patient. By this time, patient had hives on the skin of his abdomen. The resident ordered epinephrine 0.5 mL of a 1: 1000 aqueous solution subcutaneously into the upper arm and normal saline 500 mL over 30 min. He also requested the respiratory therapist to start continuous nebulized albuterol 10 mg for 1 h to address bronchospasm. Patient was also treated with diphenhydramine 25 mg IV and cimetidine 300 mg IV. With these interventions, patient had significant improvement in his symptoms, and his vital signs normalized. The resident also ordered Hydrocortisone 100 mg IV.

Debriefing

All team members agreed that communication between team members was clear and effective. All team members understood their roles and responsibilities. Situational awareness was appropriately maintained. Workload was distributed efficiently. Assistance was asked for and offered when needed. No errors were identified.

Case V

Thirty-eight-year-old female with advanced multiple sclerosis, bedbound due to paralysis, and trach and PEG-tube dependence was hospitalized due to recurrent aspiration pneumonia. She was started on appropriate antibiotics. She developed sudden onset of shortness of breath and increased work of breathing. Vital signs were remarkable for heart rate of 110, respiration rate of 28, and SpO_2 decreased to 84%. The nurse activated rapid response and started patient on continuous pulse oximetry and cardiac monitoring and applied high flow oxygen to face and the site of trach.

The ICU nurse responded immediately and assessed the patient. Patient had a chest rise and rhonchi on auscultation. The ICU nurse removed the inner cannula but was not able to pass the suction catheter; therefore, the cuff was deflated to allow extra room for the patient to ventilate on her own. Patient did not improve; therefore, the trach was removed and replaced with a smaller diameter tracheostomy tube using a bougie. With this intervention, patient was able to breath and her vital signs improved.

Debriefing

All team members agreed that communication between team members was clear and effective. All team members understood their roles and responsibilities. Situational awareness was appropriately maintained. Workload was distributed efficiently. Assistance was asked for and offered when needed. No errors were identified.

INDEX

A

Abdominal wall hematoma, 202
Accidental decanulation
  actions, 186–187
  presentation, 186
Accidental dislodgement/decannulation
  actions, 181
  causes, 181
  presentation, 181
Acquired immune deficiency syndrome (AIDS),
  170
Acute adrenal crisis
  diagnostic work-up, 107
  initial measures, 107
  presentation, 107
  symptoms, 107
Acute blood transfusion reaction
  acute hemolytic reactions, 131–132
  anaphylactic reaction, 129–130
  febrile nonhemolytic reaction, 121–122
  transfusion associated circulatory overload
    (TACO), 125–126
  transfusion-related acute lung injury, 127–128
Acute chest syndrome
  diagnostic work-up, 138–139
  initial measures, 138
  presentation, 136
  symptoms, 138
  treatment, 138
Acute complete upper airway obstruction
  diagnostic work-up, 49–50
  initial measures, 49
  presentation, 49
  symptoms, 49
  treatment, 51
Acute coronary syndrome
  diagnostic work-up, 6
  initial measures, 6
  presentation, 6
  symptoms, 6
  treatment, 6–7
Acute decompensated heart failure (ADHF)
  diagnostic work-up, 3
  initial measures, 3
  presentation, 3
  symptoms, 3
  treatment, 4
Acute hemolytic reactions
  diagnostic work-up, 131–132
  initial measures, 131

Acute hemolytic reactions *(Continued)*
  presentation, 129
  symptoms, 131
  treatment, 131
Acute hemorrhagic stroke
  diagnostic work-up, 66
  initial measures, 66
  presentation, 66
  symptoms, 66
  treatment, 66–68
Acute hyperviscosity syndrome
  diagnostic work-up, 155
  initial measures, 155
  presentation, 155
  symptoms, 155
  treatment, 156
Acute infectious diarrheal illness
  diagnostic work-up, 169–170
  initial measures, 169
  presentation, 169
  treatment, 170–171
Acute ischemic stroke
  diagnostic work-up, 63
  initial measures, 63
  presentation, 63
  symptoms, 63
  treatment, 63–65
Acute liver failure
  diagnostic work-up, 89
  initial measures, 88–89
  presentation, 88
  symptoms, 88
  treatment, 89–91
Acute pancreatitis
  diagnostic work-up, 92–93
  initial measures, 92
  presentation, 92
  treatment, 93–94
Acute partial upper airway obstruction
  diagnostic work-up, 47
  initial measures, 47
  presentation, 47
  symptoms, 47
  treatment, 48
Acute pericarditis
  diagnostic work-up, 19
  initial measures, 19
  presentation, 19
  symptoms, 19
  treatment, 20

Acute pulmonary arterial hypertension
  diagnostic work-up, 53
  initial measures, 53
  presentation, 53
  symptoms, 53
  treatment, 54
Acute respiratory distress syndrome (ARDS)
  actions, 34–35
  diagnostic work-up, 34
  presentation, 34
  symptoms, 23
  treatment, 34–35
Acute respiratory failure
  COVID-19 pneumonia, 175–177
  influenza virus infection, 172–174
  severe pneumonia, 166–168
Addisonian crisis. *See* Acute adrenal crisis
American Epilepsy Society's 2016
      guidelines, 62
American Society of Hematology (ASH), 133
American Thoracic Society and Infectious Diseases
      Society of America (ATS/IDSA) 2019
      guidelines, 166
Anaphylactic reaction
  diagnostic work-up, 129–130
  initial measures, 129
  presentation, 127
  treatment, 129
Anaphylactoid reactions
  actions, 198–199
  presentation, 198
  symptoms, 198
Anaphylaxis
  initial measures, 56
  presentation, 56
  symptoms, 56
  treatment, 56–57
Angioedema
  diagnostic work-up, 58
  presentation, 58
  symptoms, 58
  treatment, 58–59
Antipsychotics, 72
Aortic dissection
  diagnostic work-up, 18
  initial measures, 17
  presentation, 17
  symptoms, 17
  treatment, 18
Arteriovenous fistula, 196
Aspiration pneumonitis
  diagnostic work-up, 29
  initial measures, 29
  predisposing conditions, 29

Aspiration pneumonitis *(Continued)*
  presentation, 29
  treatment, 30
Asthma exacerbation
  diagnostic work-up, 23–24
  initial measures, 23
  presentation, 23
  symptoms, 23
  treatment, 24
Atelectasis
  diagnostic work-up, 39
  initial measures, 39
  presentation, 39
  symptoms, 39
  treatment, 39–40
Atrial fibrillation with rapid ventricular response
  diagnostic work-up, 10
  initial measures, 10
  presentation, 3
  symptoms, 10
  treatment, 10–12
Atypical hemolytic uremic syndrome, 144–145

B
Beta-blockers, 104
Blockage of the tracheostomy tube
  actions, 184
  presentation, 184
Bronchospasm, 197

C
Cardiac catheterization complications
  anaphylactoid reactions, 198–199
  contrast-induced nephropathy, 194–195
  hematoma, 192
  pseudoaneurysm, 196–197
  retroperitoneal hematoma, 193
Cardiac emergencies
  acute coronary syndrome, 6–7
  acute decompensated heart failure
      (ADHF), 3–5
  acute pericarditis, 19–20
  atrial fibrillation, 10–12
  cardiac tamponade, 21–22
  cardiogenic shock, 8–9
  hypertensive emergency
      acute aortic dissection, 17–18
      encephalopathy, 13–14
      hemorrhagic stroke, 15–16
      syncope, 1–2
Cardiac tamponade
  diagnostic work-up, 21

Cardiac tamponade *(Continued)*
  initial measures, 21
  presentation, 21
  symptoms, 21
  treatment, 22
Cardiogenic shock
  causes, 8
  diagnostic work-up, 8
  initial measures, 8
  presentation, 8
  treatment, 8–9
Cerebral herniation
  actions, 216–217
  presentation, 216
  symptoms, 216
Chronic obstructive pulmonary disease (COPD)
    exacerbation
  diagnostic work-up, 26
  initial measures, 26
  precipitators, 26
  presentation, 26
  treatment, 27
Community-acquired pneumonia (CAP)
  diagnostic work-up, 166–167
  initial measures, 166
  presentation, 166
  treatment, 167–168
Contrast-induced nephropathy
  actions, 194
  presentation, 194
COVID-19 (Coronavirus Disease of 2019)
    pneumonia
  diagnostic work-up, 175
  initial measures, 175
  presentation, 175
  treatment, 176

D
Delirium
  diagnostic work-up, 71–72
  initial measures, 71
  presentation, 71
  symptoms, 71
  treatment, 72
Diabetic ketoacidosis (DKA)
  diagnostic work-up, 99
  initial measures, 99
  presentation, 99
  symptoms, 99
  treatment, 99–100
Disseminated intravascular coagulation (DIC)
  diagnostic work-up, 136–137
  initial measures, 136

Disseminated intravascular coagulation (DIC)
    (Continued)
  presentation, 134
  symptoms, 136
  treatment, 136

E
Electroencephalography (EEG), 62
Endocrine emergencies
  acute adrenal crisis, 107–108
  diabetic ketoacidosis, 99–100
  hypercalcemic crisis, 109–110
  hyperkalemia, 117–118
  hypernatremia, 113–114
  hyperosmolar hyperglycemic state, 101–102
  hyperthyroidism, 103–104
  hypocalcemic crisis, 111–112
  hypokalemia, 119–120
  hyponatremia, 115–116
  hypothryroidism, 105–106
Epilepsy Foundation working group, 61

F
Facial/laryngeal edema, 197
Febrile neutropenia
  diagnostic work-up, 153
  initial measures, 153
  presentation, 153
  treatment, 153–154
Febrile nonhemolytic reaction
  diagnostic work-up, 121–122
  initial measures, 121
  presentation, 121
  treatment, 122
Femoral artery occlusion, 196
Femoral artery pseudoaneurysm, 196

G
Gastrointestinal emergencies
  acute liver failure, 88–91
  ischemic colitis, 95–96
  lower gastrointestinal bleeding, 85–87
  mesenteric ischemia, 97–98
  pancreatitis, 92–94
  upper gastrointestinal bleeding, 83–84
Graves' disease, 104
Guillain-Barre syndrome
  diagnostic work-up, 76–77
  initial measures, 76
  presentation, 76
  symptoms, 76
  treatment, 77–78

H

Headaches, 213
Hematologic emergencies
  acute chest syndrome, 138–139
  acute hemolytic reactions, 131–132
  anaphylactic reaction, 129–130
  disseminated intravascular coagulation (DIC),
    136–137
  febrile nonhemolytic reaction, 121–122
  hemolytic uremic syndrome (HUS), 144–145
  heparin-induced thrombocytopenia (HIT), 133–135
  immune thrombocytopenia (ITP), 140–141
  thrombotic thrombocytopenic purpura (TTP),
    142–143
  transfusion associated circulatory overload
    (TACO), 125–126
  transfusion-related acute lung injury, 127–128
  urticarial allergic reaction, 123–124
Hematoma
  actions, 192
  presentation, 192
  symptoms, 192
Hemolytic uremic syndrome (HUS)
  diagnostic work-up, 144–145
  initial measures, 144
  presentation, 142
  symptoms, 144
  treatment, 144
Hemoptysis, 31
Hemorrhage
  actions, 202–203
  presentation, 202
Hemorrhagic stroke
  diagnostic work-up, 15
  initial measures, 15
  presentation, 15
  treatment, 16
Hemothorax
  actions, 208
  presentation, 208
  symptoms, 208
Heparin-induced thrombocytopenia (HIT)
  diagnostic work-up, 133–134
  initial measures, 133
  presentation, 131–132
  symptoms, 133
  treatment, 133
Hepatic encephalopathy, 88
Hepatic injuries. *See* Liver and spleen injuries
Hypercalcemic crisis
  diagnostic work-up, 109–110
  initial measures, 109
  presentation, 109
  symptoms, 109

Hyperkalemia
  diagnostic work-up, 117
  initial measures, 117
  presentation, 117
  treatment, 118
Hypernatremia
  diagnostic work-up, 113
  initial measures, 113
  presentation, 113
  symptoms, 113
  treatment, 114
Hyperosmolar hyperglycemic state
  diagnostic work-up, 101
  initial measures, 101
  presentation, 101
  symptoms, 101
  treatment, 101–102
Hyperphosphatemia, 148
Hypertensive emergency, 13, 15
Hypertensive encephalopathy
  diagnostic work-up, 13
  initial measures, 13
  presentation, 13
  symptoms, 13
  treatment, 13–14
Hyperthyroidism
  diagnostic work-up, 103
  initial measures, 103
  presentation, 103
  symptoms, 103
  treatment, 104
Hypertriglyceridemia, 93
Hypocalcemic crisis
  diagnostic work-up, 111
  initial measures, 111
  presentation, 111
  symptoms, 111
  treatment, 111–112
Hypokalemia
  diagnostic work-up, 119
  initial measures, 119
  presentation, 119
  symptoms, 119
  treatment, 120
Hyponatremia
  diagnostic work-up, 115
  initial measures, 115
  presentation, 115
  symptoms, 115
  treatment, 115–116
Hypotension/shock, 197
Hypothryroidism
  diagnostic work-up, 105
  initial measures, 105

Hypothryroidism *(Continued)*
  presentation, 105
  symptoms, 105
  treatment, 105–106
Hypovolemic shock, 169–171

I

Iatrogenic empyema
  actions, 210–211
  presentation, 210
  symptoms, 210
Iatrogenic pneumothorax, 206
Idiopathic pulmonary fibrosis exacerbation
  diagnostic work-up, 51
  initial measures, 51
  presentation, 51
  symptoms, 51
  treatment, 52
Immune thrombocytopenia (ITP)
  diagnostic work-up, 140–141
  initial measures, 140
  presentation, 138
  treatment, 140
Infectious disease emergencies
  acute infectious diarrheal illness, 169–171
  community-acquired pneumonia (CAP), 166–168
  COVID-19 pneumonia, 175–177
  influenza virus infection, 172–174
  sepsis, 163–165
Inflammatory syndrome, 169
Influenza virus infection
  diagnostic work-up, 173
  initial measures, 172
  presentation, 172
  treatment, 173–174
Insulin infusion, 100–102
Intracranial hypertension
  initial measures, 69
  presentation, 69
  symptoms, 69
  treatment, 69–70
Ischemic colitis
  diagnostic work-up, 95–96
  initial measures, 95
  presentation, 95
  treatment, 96

L

Life-threatening hemoptysis
  definition, 31
  diagnostic work-up, 31
  initial measures, 31

Life-threatening hemoptysis *(Continued)*
  presentation, 31
  treatment, 31–32
Liver and spleen injuries
  actions, 212
  presentation, 212
Long-term tracheostomy complication
  accidental decanulation, 186–187
  blockage of the tracheostomy tube, 184–185
  tracheo-esophageal fistula, 188–189
  tracheo-innominate fistula, 190–191
Lower gastrointestinal bleeding
  diagnostic work-up, 86
  initial measures, 85
  presentation, 85
  symptoms, 85
  treatment, 86–87
Lumbar puncture complications
  cerebral herniation, 216–217
  post-LP headache, 213
  spinal hematoma, 214–215

M

Malignant epidural spinal cord compression
  diagnostic work-up, 159
  initial measures, 159
  presentation, 159
  symptoms, 159
  treatment, 159
Malignant pericardial effusion
  diagnostic work-up, 161
  initial measures, 161
  presentation, 161
  symptoms, 161
  treatment, 162
Massive pulmonary embolism
  diagnostic work-up, 36
  initial measures, 36
  presentation, 36
  symptoms, 36
  treatment, 36–38
Mesenteric ischemia
  diagnostic work-up, 98
  initial measures, 97
  presentation, 97
  symptoms, 97
  treatment, 98
Myasthenic crisis
  diagnostic work-up, 74
  initial measures, 74
  presentation, 74
  treatment, 75
Myxedema coma. *See* Hypothryroidism

N

National Cardiovascular Data Registry, 194
Neuroleptic malignant syndrome
  diagnostic work-up, 81–82
  initial measures, 81
  presentation, 81
  symptoms, 81
Neurological emergencies
  acute hemorrhagic stroke, 66–68
  acute ischemic stroke, 63–65
  delirium/agitation, 71–73
  Guillain-Barre syndrome, 76–78
  intracranial hypertension, 69–70
  myasthenic crisis, 74–75
  neuroleptic malignant syndrome, 81–82
  seizure/status epilepticus, 61–62
  serotonin syndrome, 79–80
Nonheparin anticoagulant, 134
Nonhistaminergic angioedema, 58
Noninflammatory syndrome, 169
Nonocclusive mesenteric ischemia, 97
Nonvariceal upper gastrointestinal bleeding, 83

O

Oncologic emergencies
  acute hyperviscosity syndrome, 155–156
  febrile neutropenia, 153–154
  malignant epidural spinal cord compression, 159–160
  malignant pericardial effusion, 161–162
  severe hypercalcemia of malignancy, 149–150
  superior vena cava syndrome, 157–158
  syndrome of inappropriate antidiuretic hormone (SIADH), 151–152
  tumor lysis syndrome, 147–148
Opioid-induced respiratory depression
  diagnostic work-up, 46
  initial measures, 45
  presentation, 45
  symptoms, 45
  treatment, 46
Oversedation, 45–46

P

Paracentesis complications
  hemorrhage, 202–203
  paracentesis-induced circulatory dysfunction, 200
  persistent leakage of ascitic fluid, 201
  visceral perforation, 204–205
Paracentesis-induced circulatory dysfunction
  actions, 200
  presentation, 200
Parathyroid hormone (PTH), 109
Partially obstructive coronary occlusion, 6

Perforation. *See* Visceral perforation
Persistent leakage of ascitic fluid
  actions, 201
  presentation, 201
Pneumothorax1. *See* Iatrogenic pneumothorax
  actions, 206–207
  presentation, 206
  symptoms, 206
Polymerase chain reaction (PCR)-based multiple
    GI pathogen panels, 170
Posterior reversible encephalopathy syndrome
    (PRES), 13
Post-LP headaches
  actions, 213
  presentation, 213
Postprocedural complications, in hospitalized
    patients
  cardiac catheterization (*see* Cardiac
    catheterization complications)
  lumbar puncture (*see* Lumbar puncture
    complications)
  paracentesis (*see* Paracentesis complications)
  thoracentesis (*see* Thoracentesis complications)
  tracheostomy
    basics, 179–180
    long-term (*see* Long-term tracheostomy
      complication)
    short-term (*see* Short-term tracheostomy
      complication)
Primary pneumothorax, 41
Pruritus, 196–197
Pseudoaneurysm
  actions, 196–197
  presentation, 196
  symptoms, 196

R

Rapid response cases
  case I, 219–220
  case II, 221
  case III, 222
  case IV, 223
  case V, 224
Respiratory emergencies
  acute hypercapnic respiratory failure, 45–46
  acute respiratory distress syndrome, 34–35
  anaphylaxis, 56–57
  aspiration pneumonitis, 29–30
  asthma exacerbation, 23–25
  atelectasis, 39–40
  complete upper airway obstruction, 49–50
  COPD exacerbation, 26–28
  idiopathic pulmonary fibrosis exacerbation, 51–52
  life-threatening hemoptysis, 31–33

Respiratory emergencies *(Continued)*
  massive pulmonary embolism, 36–38
  nonhistaminergic angioedema, 58–59
  partial upper airway obstruction, 47–48
  pulmonary arterial hypertension, 53–55
  spontaneous pneumothorax, 41–42
  tension pneumothorax, 43–44
Retroperitoneal hematoma
  actions, 193
  presentation, 193

S

Secondary spontaneous pneumothorax, 41
Seizure, 61–62
Selective serotonin reuptake inhibitors (SSRIs), 79
Sepsis
  diagnostic work-up, 164
  initial measures, 163–164
  presentation, 163
  symptoms, 163
  treatment, 164–165
Septic shock, 163–165
Sequential (sepsis-related) organ failure assessment
    (SOFA) score, 163
Serotonin syndrome
  actions, 79–80
  diagnostic work-up, 79
  presentation, 79
  symptoms, 79
  treatment, 79–80
Severe acute atelectasis. *See* Atelectasis
Severe acute pancreatitis. *See* Acute pancreatitis
Severe acute respiratory syndrome coronavirus 2
    (SARS-CoV-2), 175
Severe hypercalcemia of malignancy
  diagnostic work-up, 149
  initial measures, 149
  presentation, 149
  symptoms, 149
  treatment, 149–150
Short-term tracheostomy complication
  accidental dislodgement/decannulation, 181
  tracheostomy site hemorrhage, 182–183
Sickle cell disease, 138
Spinal hematoma
  actions, 214
  presentation, 214
  symptoms, 214
Spontaneous pneumothorax
  chronic pulmonary conditions, 41
  diagnostic work-up, 41
  initial measures, 41
  presentation, 41
  treatment, 41–42

Status asthmaticus. *See* Asthma exacerbation
Status epilepticus
  diagnostic work-up, 61–62
  initial measures, 61
  presentation, 61
  treatment, 62
Superior vena cava syndrome
  diagnostic work-up, 157
  initial measures, 157
  presentation, 157
  symptoms, 157
  treatment, 157–158
Syncope
  diagnostic work-up, 2
  initial measures, 2
  presentation, 1
  treatment, 2
  types, 1
Syndrome of inappropriate antidiuretic hormone
    (SIADH)
  diagnostic work-up, 151
  initial measures, 151
  presentation, 151
  symptoms, 151
  treatment, 151–152

T

Tension pneumothorax
  diagnostic work-up, 43
  initial measures, 43
  presentation, 43
  symptoms, 43
  treatment, 44
Thionamides, 104
Thoracentesis complications
  hemothorax, 208–209
  infection/empyema, 210–211
  liver/spleen injury, 212
  pneumothorax, 206–207
Thrombotic thrombocytopenic purpura
    (TTP)
  diagnostic work-up, 142–143
  initial measures, 142
  presentation, 140
  treatment, 142
Thyroid storm. *See* Hyperthyroidism
Tracheo-esophageal fistula
  actions, 188
  presentation, 188
  symptoms, 188
Tracheo-innominate fistula
  actions, 190–191
  presentation, 190
Tracheostomy, 179

Tracheostomy site hemorrhage
  actions, 182–183
  presentation, 182
  symptoms, 182
Transfusion associated circulatory overload
    (TACO)
  actions, 125
  presentation, 125
  symptoms, 125
Transfusion-related acute lung injury (TRALI)
  diagnostic work-up, 127–128
  initial measures, 127
  presentation, 125
  treatment, 127
Tube thoracostomy, 208
Tumor lysis syndrome
  diagnostic work-up, 147
  initial measures, 147
  presentation, 147
  treatment, 147–148

U
Upper gastrointestinal bleeding
  diagnostic work-up, 83–84
  initial measures, 83
  presentation, 83
  treatment, 84
Urticaria, 196–197
Urticarial allergic reaction
  diagnostic work-up, 123
  initial measures, 123
  presentation, 123
  symptoms, 123
  treatment, 123

V
Visceral perforation
  actions, 204–205
  presentation, 204
  symptoms, 204